HOLISTIC HEALING

HOLISTIC HEALING

Multispeciality Hospital Excellence

MARIA M

Mohammed Altaf Hussain

CONTENTS

Table of Content

Chapter 1

Introduction

All encompassing Recuperating Multispeciality Clinic Greatness: A Zenith of Far reaching Medical care

In the unique scene of contemporary medical care, where the convergence of clinical science and all encompassing prosperity characterizes the worldview of recuperating, Comprehensive Mending Multispeciality Emergency clinic remains as a reference point of greatness. Settled at the conversion of state of the art clinical headways and an all encompassing way to deal with patient consideration, this organization is focused on rethinking the medical services insight.

At the center of Comprehensive Recuperating Multispeciality Clinic's main goal is the conviction that genuine mending includes something beyond the actual part of a patient's condition. It embraces the many-sided interaction of psyche, body, and soul, perceiving the significant association between close to home prosperity and actual wellbeing. With a resolute obligation to giving a complete medical services arrangement, this clinic separates itself as a safe-haven where the workmanship and study of recuperating join.

The ethos of All encompassing Mending Multispeciality Clinic is established in a patient-driven way of thinking, setting people at the core of each and every choice and treatment plan.

The emergency clinic's devotion to greatness is obvious in its cutting edge offices, a unit of recognized clinical experts, and an integrative methodology that combines regular medication with elective treatments. This combination establishes an amicable mending climate that tends to the different necessities of patients, recognizing the uniqueness of every person and their wellbeing process.

One of the foundations of Comprehensive Mending Multispeciality Emergency clinic's obligation to greatness lies in its group of profoundly talented and humane medical care experts. From eminent experts in traditional medication to professionals of elective treatments, the clinic's multidisciplinary group teams up consistently to offer a range of medical services administrations. This combination of skill guarantees that patients get customized and balanced care, rising above the restrictions of a particular clinical methodology.

In arrangement with the clinic's comprehensive vision, All encompassing Recuperating Multispeciality Clinic invests wholeheartedly in its state of the art clinical framework. Furnished with the most recent symptomatic instruments, high level careful offices, and innovation driven therapy modalities, the emergency clinic remains at the front line of clinical development. This obligation to keeping up to date with the most recent headways guarantees that patients approach the best and productive clinical intercessions, improving the general nature of care.

Notwithstanding, All encompassing Recuperating Multispeciality Clinic perceives that genuine mending reaches out past the domain of clinical intercessions. The emergency clinic's all encompassing methodology coordinates reciprocal treatments, stressing the meaning of mental and profound prosperity in the recuperating system. From contemplation and yoga to wholesome directing and stress the board, the emergency clinic embraces a range of comprehensive modalities that enable patients to take part in their own mending process effectively.

Fundamental to the medical clinic's comprehensive way of thinking is an accentuation on preventive medical care. Perceiving the significance of proactive measures in keeping up with ideal wellbeing, All encompassing Mending Multispeciality Emergency clinic offers exhaustive wellbeing projects and wellbeing screenings. These drives point not exclusively to analyze and treat existing circumstances yet additionally to engage people with the information and apparatuses to forestall future wellbeing challenges.

Comprehensive Mending Multispeciality Medical clinic's obligation to greatness is additionally highlighted by its patient-driven way to deal with administration conveyance. The medical clinic focuses on open correspondence, encouraging a cooperative connection between medical care suppliers and patients. This approach guarantees that patients are dynamic accomplices in their medical care choices, advancing a feeling of strengthening and commitment to the mending system.

Past the walls of the clinic, Comprehensive Mending Multispeciality Medical clinic stretches out its effect on the local area through outreach programs, wellbeing training drives, and associations with nearby associations. By effectively adding to local area wellbeing and prosperity, the clinic looks to make an expanding influence of positive change, rising above individual patient consideration to have an enduring effect on the more extensive cultural wellbeing scene.

1.1 Definition of Holistic Healing

All encompassing Mending: A Thorough Investigation of Completeness in Wellbeing

All encompassing mending is an integrative way to deal with medical care that thinks about the aggregate of an individual — psyche, body, and soul — perceiving the interconnectedness of these aspects chasing after ideal wellbeing. At its center, all encompassing recuperating goes past the customary model of treating side effects and infirmities; all things being equal, it embraces a more extensive viewpoint that recognizes the intricate exchange of different elements adding to a singular's prosperity.

The underpinning of all encompassing recuperating lies in the conviction that the human body is a dynamic and interconnected framework, where actual wellbeing, mental prosperity, and otherworldly concordance are complicatedly connected. Not at all like customary clinical methodologies that frequently compartmentalize various parts of wellbeing, comprehensive mending sees the person overall substance, understanding that awkward nature in one region can appear as side effects in another. This far reaching viewpoint highlights the significance of tending to the side effects of a sickness as well as its fundamental causes, cultivating a more profound degree of mending.

In the domain of comprehensive mending, the expression "all encompassing" itself alludes to the thought of the entire individual, enveloping their physical, close to home, mental, and profound aspects. Every one of these aspects is viewed as reliant, with impacts and collaborations that shape a singular's general wellbeing. The all encompassing methodology perceives that accomplishing and keeping up with prosperity requires an agreeable equilibrium inside and between these aspects.

Actually, all encompassing mending recognizes the body's natural capacity to recuperate itself when furnished with the right circumstances. It embraces a scope of traditional clinical works on, including diagnostics, drugs, and careful mediations, however goes past these by incorporating integral and elective treatments. From needle therapy and home grown medication to rub treatment and nourishing advising, all encompassing recuperating use assorted modalities to help the body's normal mending systems.

Inwardly, comprehensive mending perceives the significant effect of mental and close to home states on actual wellbeing. Stress, tension, and irritating intense subject matters can appear as actual side effects, and addressing these hidden profound variables is fundamental to comprehensive prosperity. Restorative methodologies like guiding, psychotherapy, and stress the board procedures assume a pivotal part in reestablishing close to home equilibrium and advancing by and large wellbeing.

Intellectually, comprehensive mending envelops mental parts of wellbeing, including thought examples, convictions, and outlook. The force of the brain in impacting actual wellbeing is a focal precept of all encompassing mending. Practices like care, contemplation, and mental conduct methods are utilized to develop a positive mental climate, cultivating flexibility and adding to the counteraction and the executives of different medical issue.

Profoundly, all encompassing recuperating perceives the singular's association with a more extensive feeling of direction or importance. While not really lined up with a particular strict teaching, profound prosperity in comprehensive mending alludes to a feeling of inward harmony, reason, and association with an option that could be more significant than oneself. Rehearses that help profound prosperity might incorporate reflection, petition, or participating in exercises that bring a feeling of satisfaction and arrangement with one's qualities.

The all encompassing mending worldview reaches out past the person to think about their more extensive climate, including social, social, and biological variables. Perceiving that wellbeing is impacted by friendly help, social setting, and the soundness of the planet, all encompassing recuperating energizes a more broad perspective on wellbeing that rises above individual worries. This mindfulness stresses the significance of establishing a steady and sustaining outside climate to supplement the interior endeavors towards all encompassing prosperity.

One of the crucial standards of all encompassing mending is the emphasis on counteraction as opposed to simply treating existing circumstances. All encompassing professionals underline the significance of way of life factors, including diet, exercise, and stress the board, as primary components of keeping up with wellbeing. By tending to these viewpoints proactively, people can lessen the gamble of creating different medical problems and improve their general personal satisfaction.

All encompassing recuperating isn't expected to supplant customary medication but instead to supplement it. The joining of both traditional and elective methodologies takes into consideration a more extensive and individualized treatment plan. This joint effort between various modalities is known as integrative medication, where the qualities of each approach are utilized to advance patient consideration. This cooperative energy guarantees that people get the best and balanced medical care arrangements custom fitted to their special necessities.

In all encompassing recuperating, the patient is a functioning member in their own mending process. Engaging people with information about their wellbeing, including them in dynamic cycles, and empowering way of life adjustments are fundamental parts of the comprehensive methodology. This cooperative connection between medical services suppliers and patients cultivates a feeling of responsibility and organization, adding to the general progress of the mending system.

Comprehensive mending isn't restricted to a particular clinical strength or discipline however is a way of thinking that can be applied across different medical services settings. All encompassing standards are incorporated into the acts of medical services experts from different fields, including naturopathy, customary medication, nursing, brain science, and that's only the tip of the iceberg. This interdisciplinary methodology considers a rich embroidery of points of view, making a comprehensive medical care environment that tends to the diverse idea of human wellbeing.

1.2 Significance of a Multispeciality Hospital

The Meaning of a Multispeciality Medical clinic: An Extensive Way to deal with Medical services Greatness

In the consistently developing scene of medical care, the meaning of a multispeciality emergency clinic couldn't possibly be more significant. These establishments address a change in perspective in the conveyance of clinical benefits, offering an exhaustive and coordinated way to deal with patient consideration that goes past the bounds of customary clinical claims to fame. A multispeciality clinic, by definition, unites a different exhibit of clinical experts and particular divisions under one rooftop, making a medical care environment that takes special care of the complex necessities of patients.

At the core of the meaning of a multispeciality clinic lies the capacity to give a wide range of medical care administrations inside a bound together structure. Not at all like single-specialty emergency clinics that emphasis solely on a specific clinical discipline, multispeciality medical clinics house a scope of clinical strengths, considering a more comprehensive and cooperative way to deal with patient consideration. This inclusivity guarantees that people get complete and composed medical services, tending to both everyday practice and complex clinical requirements.

One of the vital benefits of a multispeciality clinic is the openness to an expansive range of clinical mastery inside a solitary organization. This takes out the requirement for patients to explore various medical services offices and subject matter experts, smoothing out the demonstrative and therapy process. Whether it's standard checkups, specific counsels, or crisis care, patients can track down a large number of administrations under one rooftop, working with a consistent and incorporated medical services insight.

The multidisciplinary idea of a multispeciality emergency clinic cultivates joint effort among medical services experts from different claims to fame. This cooperative model upgrades the nature of patient consideration by advancing a common perspective of individual cases and working with interdisciplinary counsels. The capacity to draw on the skill of experts from various fields guarantees that patients benefit from a balanced and informed way to deal with finding and treatment.

In the domain of preventive medical care, multispeciality clinics assume a urgent part in offering far reaching wellbeing projects and wellbeing screenings. These projects are intended to distinguish potential medical problems at a beginning phase, empowering ideal intercessions and preventive measures. From cardiovascular screenings to disease screenings and way of life directing, multispeciality clinics take a proactive position in advancing wellbeing and prosperity, adding to the general strength of the local area they serve.

The meaning of a multispeciality clinic is additionally highlighted by its ability to deal with a great many ailments and crises. With divisions committed to different clinical strengths like cardiology, muscular health, nervous system science, and the sky is the limit from there, these medical clinics are prepared to address assorted wellbeing challenges. This flexibility is particularly vital in crisis circumstances where quick admittance to specific consideration can have an effect in persistent results.

Notwithstanding clinical fortes, multispeciality emergency clinics frequently incorporate high level analytic and imaging offices. Best in class hardware, for example, X-ray, CT outputs, and research center administrations, considers exact and ideal diagnostics. This coordinated way to deal with diagnostics upholds medical care experts in pursuing informed choices and fitting therapy plans to the particular necessities of every patient.

The meaning of a multispeciality clinic reaches out past the domain of actual wellbeing to incorporate mental and profound prosperity. Numerous multispeciality clinics house divisions committed to psychological wellness, offering types of assistance like psychiatry, brain science, and directing. This acknowledgment of the psyche body association mirrors an all encompassing way to deal with medical care, recognizing that emotional well-being is an essential part of in general prosperity.

Patient-focused care is a sign of multispeciality clinics, underlining the significance of tending to the clinical requirements of patients as well as their singular inclinations and concerns. The coordination of patient-driven rehearses, for example, customized care plans, shared navigation, and patient instruction, adds to a more empathetic and enabling medical services insight. This approach cultivates a feeling of trust and organization between medical services suppliers and patients, improving the general nature of care.

With regards to ongoing and complex ailments, multispeciality clinics offer an unmistakable benefit by giving facilitated and nonstop consideration. Patients with various medical problems frequently require the mastery of experts from various fields, and a multispeciality emergency clinic smoothes out the coordination of these administrations. This cooperative model guarantees that patients with constant circumstances get far reaching and incorporated care, tending to the interconnected idea of their wellbeing challenges.

Schooling and exploration are vital parts of the meaning of a multispeciality medical clinic. These establishments frequently act as center points for clinical instruction, preparing the up and coming age of medical care experts across different claims to fame. Moreover, numerous multispeciality emergency clinics effectively participate in research exercises, adding to the progression of clinical information and the improvement of creative medicines. This obligation to schooling and examination upgrades the general nature of medical care and positions multispeciality emergency clinics as pioneers in clinical development.

The meaning of a multispeciality medical clinic isn't bound to the walls of the establishment yet reaches out to its job in local area wellbeing. These medical clinics frequently participate in local area outreach programs, wellbeing training drives, and associations with nearby associations. By effectively taking part in local area wellbeing and prosperity, multispeciality emergency clinics add to the anticipation of sicknesses, wellbeing mindfulness, and the general upgrade of general wellbeing.

1.3 Overview of Holistic Healthcare Approach

Outline of Comprehensive Medical care Approach: Sustaining Psyche, Body, and Soul

In the perplexing embroidery of medical services, the comprehensive methodology remains as a significant and enveloping way of thinking that rises above the regular limits of clinical practice. All encompassing medical services, frequently alluded to as integrative or correlative medication, perceives the perplexing transaction between the psyche, body, and soul chasing after ideal wellbeing. This comprehensive point of view recognizes that a singular's prosperity is a result of the unique interconnection of different factors, and genuine mending includes tending to the entirety of an individual's being.

At the core of the all encompassing medical care approach is the conviction that the human body has inborn mending components. Instead of only treating side effects, all encompassing experts endeavor to help and upgrade the body's inherent capacity to recuperate itself. This basic rule lines up with the old insight of numerous customary recuperating frameworks, where the accentuation is put on reestablishing harmony and congruity inside the person.

The comprehensive model perceives that actual wellbeing is unpredictably associated with close to home and mental prosperity.

Stress, for instance, is recognized as a critical supporter of different medical problems, and comprehensive medical services tries to address the main drivers of stress, consolidating modalities like unwinding methods, reflection, and care to advance close to home and mental balance. This interconnected point of view accentuates that close to home and mental states can significantly affect actual wellbeing as well as the other way around.

From an actual outlook, all encompassing medical care coordinates regular clinical practices with a horde of reciprocal and elective treatments. Ordinary medication, with its symptomatic devices, drug mediations, and surgeries, is supplemented by all encompassing modalities, for example, needle therapy, home grown medication, chiropractic care, and wholesome directing. This coordination makes a far reaching and individualized way to deal with patient consideration, perceiving that every individual is one of a kind and may profit from a different scope of helpful intercessions.

Nourishment assumes a significant part in the comprehensive medical care approach, seeing food as food as well as a basic part of wellbeing and recuperating. Comprehensive sustenance underlines the significance of entire, supplement thick food sources that feed the body at a cell level. Dietary proposals are customized to individual requirements, considering variables like digestion, stomach related wellbeing, and explicit medical issue. This dietary methodology reaches out past the idea of calorie building up to embrace the possibility that food is a type of medication, impacting actual wellbeing as well as mental and profound prosperity.

Comprehensive medical care perceives the meaning of avoidance and way of life changes in keeping up with ideal wellbeing. As opposed to trusting that sickness will show, the accentuation is put on proactive measures that help generally speaking prosperity. Way of life factors like standard actual work, satisfactory rest, and stress the executives are essential parts of the comprehensive methodology. By enabling people to settle on informed decisions about their way of life, all encompassing medical care tries to forestall the beginning of illnesses and advance life span.

Mental and profound aspects are key to the comprehensive medical services worldview. The psyche body association is a core value, underscoring the effect of mental states on actual wellbeing. Practices like contemplation, yoga, and care are integrated to advance mental clearness, close to home equilibrium, and a feeling of internal harmony. The otherworldly aspect, while not really lined up with a particular strict convention, recognizes the significance of interfacing with a more profound feeling of direction, importance, or greatness. This acknowledgment of otherworldliness as a part of wellbeing mirrors the all encompassing comprehension of people as multi-layered creatures.

All encompassing medical services stretches out past the bounds of individual wellbeing worries to embrace a more extensive natural viewpoint. The interconnectedness of human wellbeing with the strength of the climate is recognized, underscoring the significance of maintainable practices and ecological stewardship. This natural mindfulness lines up with the comprehension that the prosperity of people is unpredictably connected to the prosperity of the planet, cultivating a feeling of obligation for both individual and planetary wellbeing.

The comprehensive medical care approach esteems the job of the patient as a functioning member in their own mending process. As opposed to a more paternalistic model of medical care, where the medical services supplier expects a mandate job, all encompassing professionals participate in a cooperative relationship with their patients. This organization includes open correspondence, shared independent direction, and a common obligation to the standards of all encompassing consideration. Patients are engaged with data and urged to take responsibility for wellbeing, cultivating a feeling of organization and self-viability.

The comprehensive medical services model incorporates an extensive variety of medical care experts from different disciplines. Naturopathic specialists, alignment specialists, acupuncturists, nutritionists, clinicians, and back rub advisors are among the experts who add to the comprehensive medical services environment. This variety takes into consideration a rich embroidery of points of view, making a multidisciplinary approach that tends to the intricacy of human wellbeing. The cooperative idea of comprehensive medical services advances cross-disciplinary correspondence and shared information, enhancing the general nature of care.

Integrative medication is a term frequently utilized reciprocally with all encompassing medical services, featuring the joining of regular and corresponding ways to deal with patient consideration. In integrative medication, the qualities of both regular and comprehensive modalities are utilized to improve patient results. This cooperative model recognizes the worth of proof based rehearses while embracing the all encompassing comprehension of wellbeing and recuperating.

The meaning of all encompassing medical care reaches out to the domain of persistent and complex ailments. Comprehensive experts perceive that persistent circumstances frequently require a multi-layered approach, tending to the actual side effects as well as the basic causes and contributing variables. By taking into account the interconnected idea of wellbeing, all encompassing medical services offers a more complete and customized system for overseeing constant diseases, stressing way of life changes, steady treatments, and preventive measures.

Patient instruction is a foundation of the comprehensive medical services approach. Comprehensive professionals endeavor to engage their patients with information about their wellbeing, empowering them to pursue informed choices and take on way of life rehearses that help prosperity. Training reaches out past the treatment room, enveloping studios, classes, and assets that advance wellbeing education and proactive commitment to one's wellbeing.

Chapter 2

The Foundations of Holistic Healing

The Underpinnings of All encompassing Mending: Overcoming any issues Among Science and Otherworldliness

All encompassing mending, as a worldview of medical care, lays on an establishment that rises above the conventional limits of medication. At its center, all encompassing recuperating recognizes the complex transaction of different elements of human life — psyche, body, and soul — and perceives the powerful interconnectedness of these features chasing prosperity. This comprehensive methodology tries to address the side effects of an infirmity as well as the fundamental causes, taking into account the person overall substance with one of a kind physical, profound, mental, and otherworldly perspectives.

One of the central standards of comprehensive recuperating is the confidence in the body's intrinsic capacity to mend itself. This guideline lines up with the old insight of numerous customary recuperating frameworks that view the body as an automatic and self-mending organic entity.

Comprehensive experts accentuate supporting and upgrading the body's regular mending components, encouraging a climate helpful for wellbeing and prosperity. This fundamental conviction challenges the reductionist point of view that frequently overwhelms regular medication, where side effects are treated in disconnection without essentially tending to the underlying drivers.

All encompassing mending perceives the interconnected idea of actual wellbeing, mental prosperity, and close to home equilibrium. The brain body association is a focal fundamental of this worldview, recognizing that psychological and profound states can essentially impact actual wellbeing. Stress, for instance, is perceived as a contributing element to different medical problems, and comprehensive mending looks to address pressure through modalities like contemplation, unwinding methods, and care. This integrative viewpoint highlights the significance of thinking about the entire individual chasing wellbeing.

The all encompassing model perspectives wellbeing not simply as the shortfall of infection but rather as a condition of dynamic equilibrium and congruity inside the person. This viewpoint goes past the reductionist methodology of recognizing and treating explicit side effects and dives into the more extensive setting of a singular's general prosperity. The accentuation is put on preventive measures, way of life alterations, and proactive methodologies that help ideal wellbeing and forestall the beginning of illnesses. All encompassing mending welcomes people to effectively take part in their wellbeing process, cultivating a feeling of obligation and strengthening.

Nourishment assumes a significant part in the underpinnings of all encompassing recuperating, perceiving that food isn't just a wellspring of food yet a central part of wellbeing. All encompassing nourishment stresses the significance of entire, supplement thick food varieties that furnish the body with the vital structure blocks for ideal working. Dietary proposals are customized to individual necessities, considering variables like metabolic rate, stomach related wellbeing, and explicit medical issue. This wholesome methodology reaches out past the idea of diets and calorie counting, embracing that food is a type of medication that impacts actual wellbeing as well as mental and profound prosperity.

The comprehensive model stretches out past the person to include the more extensive social and natural setting. Social determinants of wellbeing, like admittance to instruction, financial status, and local area support, are recognized as variables that influence a singular's prosperity. All encompassing recuperating perceives the significance of establishing a steady outside climate that supplements the inward endeavors towards wellbeing. This biological viewpoint likewise stretches out to the planet, underscoring economical practices and natural stewardship as necessary parts of all encompassing prosperity.

Otherworldliness is one more central component of all encompassing recuperating, in spite of the fact that it isn't really lined up with a particular strict teaching. All things being equal, otherworldliness in the comprehensive setting alludes to a more profound feeling of significance, reason, and association with an option that could be more significant than oneself. This otherworldly aspect perceives that people might view as mending and comfort through rehearses that line up with their own convictions, whether through supplication, reflection, or commitment to exercises that cultivate a feeling of greatness. The acknowledgment of otherworldliness as a part of wellbeing mirrors the comprehensive comprehension of people as complex creatures.

All encompassing recuperating additionally accentuates the meaning of energy stream inside the body. Numerous conventional recuperating frameworks, like Customary Chinese Medication and Ayurveda, perceive the presence of energy pathways or channels. In these frameworks, disturbances in the progression of energy are accepted to add to sickness, and helpful modalities like needle therapy, pressure point massage, and energy recuperating expect to reestablish harmony and amicability. While the idea of energy stream might be less natural in ordinary clinical settings, it is fundamental to numerous all encompassing practices.

Care and contemplation are vital parts of the all encompassing mending approach. These practices, established in old scrutinizing customs, are perceived for their capacity to advance mental lucidity, profound equilibrium, and a feeling of inward harmony. Care includes developing present-second mindfulness, permitting people to notice their contemplations and sentiments without connection or judgment. Contemplation, then again, includes various procedures that advance unwinding, focus, and mindfulness. Both care and contemplation add to the comprehensive model by tending to the psychological and close to home elements of wellbeing.

The comprehensive mending worldview reaches out past the limits of individual medical care practices to include a different cluster of medical services experts and modalities. Naturopathic specialists, bone and joint specialists, acupuncturists, nutritionists, knead advisors, and clinicians are among the experts who add to the all encompassing medical services environment. This variety considers a multidisciplinary approach, where alternate points of view and modalities can be coordinated to address the intricacy of human wellbeing. The cooperative idea of all encompassing medical services advances cross-disciplinary correspondence and shared information, enhancing the general nature of care.

Patient training is a foundation of the comprehensive mending approach. Comprehensive professionals endeavor to engage their patients with information about their wellbeing, empowering them to settle on informed choices and take on way of life rehearses that help prosperity. Training reaches out past the treatment room, enveloping studios, workshops, and assets that advance wellbeing education and proactive commitment to one's wellbeing. This instructive part mirrors the all encompassing model's obligation to cultivating a feeling of organization and self-viability in people.

Integrative medication is a term frequently utilized reciprocally with comprehensive recuperating, featuring the joining of ordinary and corresponding ways to deal with patient consideration. In integrative medication, the qualities of both regular and comprehensive modalities are utilized to streamline patient results. This cooperative model recognizes the worth of proof based rehearses while embracing the all encompassing comprehension of wellbeing and recuperating. Integrative medication is earning respect in standard medical services settings, mirroring a developing affirmation of the all encompassing model's viability.

Research in the field of all encompassing mending is an advancing undertaking, with a rising spotlight on investigating the viability of different correlative and elective treatments. While comprehensive practices frequently draw on conventional insight and episodic proof, there is a developing interest in exposing these modalities to thorough logical examination. Research concentrates on care based mediations, needle therapy, home grown medication, and other comprehensive methodologies add to the proof base supporting the all encompassing mending worldview. This convergence of customary thinking and logical request mirrors a scaffold between the natural and exact parts of medical care.

2.1 Historical Perspectives on Holistic Medicine

Verifiable Viewpoints on Comprehensive Medication: Following the Underlying foundations of a Groundbreaking Worldview

The idea of comprehensive medication, frequently alluded to as all encompassing recuperating or integrative medication, has profound authentic roots that length societies, customs, and hundreds of years. While the expression "comprehensive medication" itself might be generally present day, the standards basic this worldview have been woven into the texture of different recuperating customs over the entire course of time. This investigation digs into the verifiable points of view that established the groundwork for the comprehensive medication we perceive today, following its development through time and across different societies.

Antiquated Recuperating Customs:

The underlying foundations of comprehensive medication can be followed back to old mending customs that saw wellbeing as a condition of equilibrium and concordance inside the individual and the climate. In old China, Conventional Chinese Medication (TCM) arose as a comprehensive framework that enveloped needle therapy, home grown medication, rub (tui na), and practices like qigong. TCM underscored the idea of Qi, the indispensable energy that moves through the body, and tried to keep up with the harmony between Yin and Yang powers.

Likewise, Ayurveda, the old recuperating arrangement of India, goes back more than 5,000 years and is grounded in an all encompassing comprehension of wellbeing.

Ayurveda sees people as extraordinary mixes of the three doshas — Vata, Pitta, and Kapha — and looks to orchestrate these doshas to advance prosperity. Dietary practices, natural cures, and way of life changes are necessary to Ayurvedic medication, mirroring an all encompassing methodology that addresses physical, mental, and otherworldly aspects.

The old Greeks additionally added to the groundworks of all encompassing medication. Hippocrates, frequently viewed as the dad of Western medication, underscored the significance of treating the entire individual instead of simply the side effects. His well known expression, "Let food be thy endlessly medication be thy food," highlights the all encompassing viewpoint that perceives the job of diet and way of life in keeping up with wellbeing.

Customary Recuperating Practices:

As civilizations prospered, various societies all over the planet fostered their own conventional recuperating rehearses established in comprehensive standards. Local American medication, for example, frequently consolidated profound ceremonies, home grown cures, and a profound association with nature. Local healers perceived the interconnectedness of physical, mental, and profound prosperity, seeing wellbeing as an impression of congruity with the normal world.

In Africa, conventional recuperating frameworks changed across districts yet generally coordinated profound practices, home grown medication, and local area support. The comprehensive methodology in African conventional medication stretched out past individual wellbeing to envelop shared prosperity, stressing the significance of social agreement and equilibrium.

Recovery of Comprehensive Thoughts in the West:

While comprehensive standards endured in different conventional recuperating frameworks, the Western world encountered a shift toward reductionism and specialization during the Renaissance and the Time of Edification. The logical upset achieved huge headways in figuring out the human body and sickness, prompting the improvement of current medication. While these improvements contributed gigantically to clinical information and innovation, they likewise encouraged a reductionist worldview that frequently compartmentalized wellbeing into particular frameworks and fortes.

The nineteenth and mid twentieth hundreds of years saw a resurgence of interest in comprehensive thoughts in the West. The psyche body association acquired consideration, and the effect of mental and close to home states on actual wellbeing turned into a subject of investigation. Trailblazers like Florence Songbird, a central figure in nursing, underscored the significance of all encompassing consideration and the job of the climate in recuperating.

Comprehensive Developments in the twentieth Hundred years:

The mid-twentieth century denoted an outstanding resurgence of all encompassing thoughts, catalyzed by people and developments that tried to reintegrate the divided parts of medical services. One such powerful figure was Sir William Osler, a conspicuous doctor in the late nineteenth and mid twentieth hundreds of years. Osler upheld for a more persistent focused and caring way to deal with medication, perceiving the singularity of patients and the significance of grasping their lives with regards to wellbeing.

The comprehensive wellbeing development picked up speed during the 1960s and 1970s, energized by social movements, disappointment with the limits of ordinary medication, and a developing interest in elective mending modalities. Rachel Carson's weighty book, "Quiet Spring," caused to notice ecological issues and the interconnectedness of human wellbeing with the strength of the planet. This biological mindfulness lined up with all encompassing standards, underscoring the significance of a reasonable and practical climate for prosperity.

Mind-Body Medication and All encompassing Practices:

The last 50% of the twentieth century saw the rise of psyche body medication as a noticeable field inside comprehensive medical care. Trailblazers like Dr. Herbert Benson investigated the physiological impacts of reflection and unwinding strategies, featuring the impact of mental states on actual wellbeing. The brain body association turned into a point of convergence, with practices like contemplation, yoga, and biofeedback earning respect for their remedial advantages.

Comprehensive practices, for example, needle therapy, chiropractic care, and home grown medication, which had establishes in antiquated customs, acquired prominence in the West during this period. Needle therapy, a fundamental part of Customary

Chinese Medication, earned revenue for its viability in tending to a scope of ailments. Chiropractic care, established by D.D. Palmer in the late nineteenth 100 years, zeroed in on the connection between spinal wellbeing and by and large prosperity. Home grown medication, drawing on the insight of conventional recuperating frameworks, encountered a restoration as people looked for normal options in contrast to drug mediations.

Arrangement of Comprehensive Organizations:

The last option a piece of the twentieth century likewise saw the foundation of establishments devoted to all encompassing medical services and examination. The American Comprehensive Clinical Affiliation (AHMA), established in 1978, planned to advance the standards of all encompassing medication and give a stage to cooperation among all encompassing specialists. The foundation of all encompassing focuses and instructive projects additionally added to the systematization of comprehensive standards inside the medical care scene.

Reconciliation into Standard Medical care:

The 21st century saw a prominent shift as all encompassing thoughts incorporated into standard medical services. Integrative medication, a methodology that joins ordinary and reciprocal treatments, earned respect as significant clinical organizations laid out integrative medication offices. The Consortium of Scholarly Wellbeing Places for Integrative Medication, shaped in 1999, epitomizes the developing cooperation between traditional clinical establishments and comprehensive experts.

Significant clinical focuses began consolidating comprehensive modalities like needle therapy, rub treatment, and care into patient consideration. Research on correlative and elective treatments picked up speed, adding to the proof base supporting the adequacy of comprehensive methodologies. This joining mirrors a more comprehensive medical services worldview that recognizes the worth of different recuperating modalities in tending to the mind boggling necessities of patients.

Difficulties and Open doors:

While comprehensive medication has acquired acknowledgment, it keeps on confronting difficulties and suspicion inside specific fragments of the clinical local area. A few pundits contend that the absence of normalized rehearses and the variety of all encompassing modalities present difficulties in laying out a brought together logical establishment. Others express worries about the potential for falsehood and problematic medicines inside the domain of all encompassing medical services.

Notwithstanding, the continuous investigation of all encompassing standards and practices presents open doors for a more nuanced and patient-focused way to deal with medical services. The ascent of customized medication, which tailors treatment plans to individual hereditary, ecological, and way of life factors, lines up with all encompassing standards. The acknowledgment of social determinants of wellbeing and the significance of emotional wellness in generally prosperity further line up with the comprehensive worldview.

2.2 Evolution of Multispeciality Hospitals

The idea of multispeciality clinics addresses a critical development in the scene of medical services, denoting a takeoff from the conventional model of single-specialty establishments. The development of multispeciality emergency clinics is a demonstration of the dynamic and complex nature of medical care needs, as well as the acknowledgment that a more complete and coordinated approach is fundamental for tending to the different wellbeing challenges looked by people. This investigation follows the verifiable turn of events and key achievements in the development of multispeciality emergency clinics, revealing insight into the variables that have formed their development and unmistakable quality in the contemporary medical services scene.

Authentic Roots:

The underlying foundations of multispeciality care can be followed back to the late nineteenth and mid twentieth hundreds of years when emergency clinics basically centered around broad medication and medical procedure. As clinical information progressed, fortes started to arise, prompting the foundation of particular emergency clinics taking care of explicit clinical disciplines. Notwithstanding, the constraints of this particular model became clear as patients with different medical problems required care from different subject matter experts.

The shift towards multispeciality care picked up speed during the twentieth 100 years. With the acknowledgment that people frequently gave intricate and interconnected medical problems, the requirement for a more planned and cooperative methodology became clear. The development of innovation, symptomatic progressions, and the developing intricacy of clinical medicines additionally accentuated the need of uniting experts from different disciplines under one rooftop.

Progressions in Clinical Strengths:

The development of multispeciality clinics has been firmly entwined with headways in clinical strengths. As clinical information extended, new claims to fame arose, each zeroing in on a particular organ framework, sickness class, or patient segment. Cardiology, nervous system science, muscular health, oncology, and other particular fields fostered their own aptitude and advances, adding to the general intricacy of medical services.

These particular fields, while essential for top to bottom comprehension and treatment of explicit circumstances, featured the requirement for cooperation and coordination in persistent consideration. Patients with numerous medical problems frequently required the mastery of various trained professionals, prompting the acknowledgment that a more all encompassing and incorporated approach was fundamental for ideal medical services conveyance.

Rise of Far reaching Care Focuses:

Because of the developing requirement for far reaching care, the mid-twentieth century saw the foundation of thorough consideration habitats that expected to give a scope of clinical benefits under one rooftop. These focuses united experts from different fields to work cooperatively in the determination, treatment, and the executives of patients. While not yet completely multispeciality emergency clinics, these focuses laid the preparation for the incorporated consideration model that would later characterize multispeciality foundations.

Mechanical Progressions and Analytic Abilities:

The last option some portion of the twentieth century saw noteworthy mechanical progressions in medical care. The improvement of modern symptomatic apparatuses, imaging advances, and lab procedures changed how sicknesses were distinguished and treated. These progressions worked on the precision of judgments as well as worked with the cooperation between various fortes by giving a more complete perspective on patients' wellbeing.

The accessibility of cutting edge symptomatic capacities assumed a significant part in the development of multispeciality emergency clinics. With the capacity to lead many demonstrative tests in-house, these medical clinics could offer a more smoothed out and productive way to deal with patient consideration. Ideal and precise diagnostics turned into a foundation of multispeciality care, considering faster navigation and more successful treatment techniques.

Changing Socioeconomics and Medical care Needs:

The switching socioeconomics of populaces up the world have additionally added to the advancement of multispeciality clinics. As populaces age, the pervasiveness of constant and complex medical issue increments. More established grown-ups frequently present with a mix of clinical issues that require the skill of experts from different fields, like cardiology, geriatrics, and muscular health.

Furthermore, the change in ways of life, ecological variables, and the ascent of non-transmittable sicknesses have prompted a more different and complex medical services scene. People are looking for care for a more extensive scope of wellbeing concerns, requiring a methodology that goes past the capacities of single-specialty establishments.

Combination of All encompassing and Preventive Consideration:

The advancement of multispeciality emergency clinics has likewise seen a rising acknowledgment of the significance of all encompassing and preventive consideration. While particular medicines for explicit circumstances are fundamental, the comprehensive methodology recognizes the interconnected idea of wellbeing. Incorporating comprehensive practices, for example, nourishment directing, emotional wellness administrations, and way of life intercessions, has turned into a sign of multispeciality care.

Preventive consideration has acquired noticeable quality as multispeciality medical clinics mean to address medical problems at their underlying foundations and lessen the weight of persistent sicknesses. Wellbeing programs, wellbeing screenings, and local area outreach drives are indispensable parts of the administrations presented by these medical clinics. This shift towards counteraction mirrors a more extensive comprehension of medical care that reaches out past getting sicknesses advancing generally speaking prosperity.

Patient-Driven Approach and Coordination of Care:

Multispeciality medical clinics are described by a patient-driven approach that underlines facilitated and customized care. The coordination of care among different strengths guarantees that patients get extensive and incorporated treatment plans. The patient's process is smoothed out, with medical care suppliers teaming up to address the quick wellbeing worries as well as the fundamental factors that might add to the patient's prosperity.

The multidisciplinary idea of multispeciality medical clinics empowers medical care groups to cooperate, sharing bits of knowledge and mastery to foster a comprehensive comprehension of the patient's wellbeing. This cooperative model cultivates correspondence among trained professionals, lessening the probability of divided care and guaranteeing that all parts of the patient's wellbeing are thought of.

Mechanical Combination and Telemedicine:

The advancement of multispeciality medical clinics has been intently attached to the combination of innovation into medical care conveyance. Electronic wellbeing records (EHRs), telemedicine, and computerized correspondence stages have changed the manner in which medical services suppliers communicate with patients and work together with one another. The consistent trade of data has upgraded the coherence of care and worked on the general patient experience.

Telemedicine, specifically, has turned into a significant part of multispeciality care, permitting patients to get to counsels and subsequent meet-ups from a distance. This has demonstrated particularly advantageous for people in far off areas, those with versatility difficulties, or those looking for expert sentiments without the requirement for broad travel. The joining of innovation has extended the scope of multispeciality clinics, making particular consideration more open to different populaces.

Difficulties and Future Bearings:

While the development of multispeciality emergency clinics has achieved critical upgrades in medical care conveyance, challenges persevere. One test is the requirement for compelling correspondence and cooperation among medical care suppliers from various claims to fame. Guaranteeing consistent coordination of care requires powerful frameworks for data trade and interdisciplinary cooperation.

One more test includes offsetting specialization with the requirement for a comprehensive and patient-driven approach. The gamble of siloed rehearses, where experts center exclusively around their subject matter disregarding the more extensive wellbeing setting, stays a worry. Endeavors to advance a culture of cooperation and interdisciplinary learning are fundamental for tending to this test.

The monetary ramifications of keeping up with multispeciality medical clinics, with different claims to fame and cutting edge innovations, present difficulties concerning asset distribution and manageability. Effective administration, key preparation, and an emphasis on streamlining functional cycles are essential for guaranteeing the financial practicality of these foundations.

Planning ahead, the development of multispeciality emergency clinics is probably going to go on because of arising medical services needs and mechanical progressions.

The coordination of man-made consciousness (computer based intelligence) and information investigation holds guarantee for improving diagnostics, treatment arranging, and customized medication. The utilization of man-made intelligence in prescient examination can assist with recognizing wellbeing chances and mediate pro-actively, lining up with the preventive consideration focal point of multispeciality emergency clinics.

The accentuation on quiet commitment and strengthening is supposed to develop, with an expanded spotlight on shared navigation and patient schooling. Engaging patients with data and including them in their consideration plans lines up with the patient-driven ethos of multispeciality emergency clinics.

The continuous advancement of multispeciality clinics additionally crosses with more extensive patterns in medical services, for example, the shift towards esteem based care and populace wellbeing the board. The accentuation on further developing wellbeing results, upgrading patient encounters, and controlling medical services costs lines up with the objectives of multispeciality care, which looks to give superior grade, composed, and productive medical care administrations.

2.3 Integration of Traditional and Modern Medicine

The combination of customary and present day medication addresses a dynamic and developing worldview in the field of medical services. Conventional medication, established in old recuperating practices, and present day medication, described by logical thoroughness and mechanical headways, have long coincided as particular ways to deal with mending. Notwithstanding, a rising acknowledgment of the reciprocal qualities of these two frameworks has prompted a developing development towards their combination. This investigation dives into the verifiable roots, philosophical establishments, difficulties, and open doors related with the coordination of custom-ary and present day medication, exhibiting how this collaboration can add to a more all encompassing and patient-focused way to deal with medical care.

Authentic Points of view:

The verifiable mix of conventional and current medication can be followed back to old civilizations where healers and specialists utilized a mix of normal cures, customs, and experimental perceptions. In old China, Customary Chinese Medication (TCM) developed as a comprehensive framework that enveloped needle therapy, home grown medication, and different psyche body rehearses. Likewise, Ayurveda, the conventional arrangement of medication in India, has a set of experiences going back millennia and is grounded in a comprehensive comprehension of wellbeing and prosperity.

As social orders advanced, the appearance of present day medication achieved criti-cal headways in logical figuring out, analytic apparatuses, and drug mediations.

The logical upset and the development of proof based medication in the nine-teenth and twentieth hundreds of years denoted a shift towards a more precise and normalized way to deal with medical services. This period saw the foundation of present day clinical organizations and the improvement of thorough philosophies for testing and approving clinical mediations.

Philosophical Establishments:

The reconciliation of customary and current medication lays on the acknowledgment that every framework carries one of a kind qualities to the medical services scene. Conventional medication frequently underlines a comprehensive methodology, seeing wellbeing as a harmony between brain, body, and soul. Practices like needle therapy, natural medication, and psyche body methods mean to reestablish congruity and address the main drivers of ailment.

Then again, present day medication is portrayed by a reductionist methodology, zeroing in on the distinguishing proof and treatment of explicit illnesses through proof based rehearses. Mechanical progressions, symptomatic accuracy, and drug mediations play had a crucial impact in the wonderful accomplishments of present day medication, particularly in regions like irresistible sicknesses, medical procedure, and crisis care.

The philosophical underpinnings of reconciliation lie in the affirmation that neither one of the frameworks is comprehensive in tending to the intricacies of medical services. Conventional medication's accentuation on anticipation, comprehensive wellbeing, and customized care lines up with the developing acknowledgment of the significance of these perspectives in present day medical care. On the other hand, present day medication's analytic capacities, logical meticulousness, and intense consideration intercessions carry important apparatuses to address complicated and intense wellbeing challenges.

Corresponding Qualities:

The incorporation of customary and present day medication exploits their corresponding assets to offer a more thorough and patient-focused way to deal with medical services. Customary medication, with its accentuation on preventive consideration and comprehensive prosperity, can add to wellbeing advancement and illness anticipation methodologies. Rehearses like yoga, contemplation, and dietary mediations from customary frameworks can assume a part in overseeing constant circumstances and advancing generally health.

Current medication, with its high level demonstrative apparatuses and proof based mediations, succeeds in intense consideration settings, crisis circumstances, and the administration of complicated sicknesses. Surgeries, drug medicines, and mechanical advancements have changed the scene of medication, empowering medical care suppliers to determine and get infections have exceptional accuracy.

The integrative methodology perceives that patients might profit from the qualities of the two frameworks, taking into consideration a more customized and nuanced treatment plan. For example, a malignant growth patient going through chemotherapy may at the same time get support from conventional medication through corresponding treatments to oversee incidental effects, upgrade prosperity, and work on personal satisfaction.

Challenges in Reconciliation:

Regardless of the expected advantages, the coordination of conventional and present day medication faces difficulties that come from contrasts in way of thinking, practice, and institutional designs. One critical test lies in overcoming any barrier between the social and philosophical differentiations of customary and present day medication. Customary medication frequently works inside a system well established in social convictions, otherworldliness, and the idea of fundamental energy, which might contrast essentially from the reductionist and materialistic perspective of present day medication.

Normalization and guideline represent extra difficulties. Customary medication envelops a different scope of practices and approaches, and guaranteeing consistency in quality and wellbeing can be perplexing. Laying out normalized rules for the joining of conventional treatments inside present day medical services systems requires cautious thought of social, moral, and wellbeing contemplations.

Another test is the shifting degrees of proof supporting conventional treatments. While numerous customary practices have exhibited viability through hundreds of years of purpose, the absence of thorough logical approval can be a boundary to their acknowledgment in current medical services settings. Incorporating customary treatments into proof based models requires powerful exploration, clinical preliminaries, and a structure for assessing the security and viability of these intercessions.

Institutional obstruction and absence of mindfulness among medical services experts can likewise block the coordination cycle. Customary medication is frequently minimized inside standard medical services frameworks, and an absence of understanding or appreciation for its worth might frustrate cooperative endeavors. Defeating these obstructions requires schooling, preparing, and a change in institutional perspectives towards a more comprehensive and all encompassing way to deal with patient consideration.

Amazing open doors for Combination:

While challenges exist, a few potential open doors can work with the consistent combination of conventional and present day medication, cultivating a more comprehensive and patient-focused medical care framework.

Exploration and Proof Structure:

Powerful logical examination is fundamental for laying out the wellbeing and viability of customary treatments. Cooperative endeavors between customary healers, specialists, and current medical services experts can add to building a proof base for conventional intercessions. This examination can assist with distinguishing explicit circumstances where conventional treatments might be best and guide the advancement of integrative treatment conventions.

Schooling and Preparing:

Coordinating conventional and present day medication requires schooling and preparing programs that overcome any issues between the two frameworks. Medical services experts ought to be outfitted with the information and abilities to comprehend and integrate conventional treatments into their training. Likewise, customary healers could profit from preparing programs that acquaint them with present day symptomatic and treatment draws near.

Social Skill:

A socially able medical services framework is urgent for fruitful joining. Understanding the social setting in which conventional medication works, regarding different conviction frameworks, and cultivating open correspondence among patients and medical care suppliers are fundamental parts of socially delicate consideration. This approach advances trust and joint effort, upgrading the viability of incorporated care.

Patient-Focused Care:

Putting patients at the focal point of their medical care experience is a major rule of coordination. Connecting with patients in shared navigation, figuring out their inclinations, and regarding their social convictions enable people to effectively take part in their treatment plans. Patient-focused care recognizes the worth of comprehensive prosperity and the significance of tending to physical, mental, and profound components of wellbeing.

Cooperative Medical services Models:

Cooperative medical services models that unite experts from both conventional and current frameworks can make collaborations that benefit patients. Integrative medical services facilities and focuses, where customary healers and present day medical services experts work next to each other, give a stage to shared information, cross-disciplinary coordinated effort, and complete patient consideration.

Government Backing and Strategy:

Government strategies that perceive and uphold the coordination of customary and present day medication are instrumental in establishing an empowering climate. Laying out administrative systems, financing research drives, and integrating integrative methodologies into public medical services techniques show a guarantee to comprehensive and comprehensive medical care rehearses.

Instances of Effective Incorporation:

A few nations have made progress in effectively coordinating conventional and current medication, giving significant instances of how this cooperative energy can be accomplished.

China:

Conventional Chinese Medication (TCM) is profoundly incorporated into China's medical care framework. TCM medical clinics and centers coincide with current clinical offices, and specialists frequently team up to offer coordinated care. The public authority has carried out arrangements to help TCM exploration, schooling, and work on, perceiving its social and restorative worth.

India:

India has a rich custom of Ayurveda, Yoga, Naturopathy, Unani, Siddha, and Homeopathy (AYUSH). The public authority has laid out the Service of

Germany:

Germany has embraced integrative medication through the foundation of facilities and focuses that offer a mix of regular and reciprocal treatments. The German Culture for Integrative Medication advocates for the joining of proof based correlative treatments inside standard medical care, encouraging a cooperative way to deal with patient consideration.

US:

In the US, integrative medication has acquired acknowledgment with the foundation of integrative medical care habitats. These focuses offer a mix of customary medicines, corresponding treatments, and way of life intercessions. Scholastic organizations have likewise evolved integrative medication programs, underlining an entire individual way to deal with medical services.

Chapter 3

The Role of Multispeciality Hospitals in Holistic Healing

The Job of Multispeciality Clinics in All encompassing Recuperating: Exploring the Range of Exhaustive Consideration

Multispeciality emergency clinics have arisen as essential players in the developing scene of medical services, offering a different scope of clinical benefits under one rooftop. Their job in comprehensive recuperating reaches out past the customary treatment of sicknesses, embracing a more extensive vision that envelops physical, mental, and profound prosperity. This investigation digs into the multi-layered job of multispeciality clinics in comprehensive recuperating, analyzing the reconciliation of different clinical claims to fame, patient-driven care, preventive measures, and the advancement of generally speaking health.

Incorporation of Assorted Clinical Fortes:

At the core of the multispeciality clinic's job in all encompassing mending is the reconciliation of different clinical fortes. Customarily, medical services conveyance was compartmentalized, with particular clinics zeroing in on unambiguous teaches like cardiology, muscular health, or nervous system science.

Multispeciality emergency clinics, in any case, unite specialists from different fields, encouraging joint effort and guaranteeing that patients get complete and facilitated care.

This reconciliation is especially important while tending to intricate and interconnected medical problems. Patients frequently present with conditions that include various organ frameworks or require the aptitude of experts from various disciplines. In a multispeciality medical clinic, these experts cooperate, sharing experiences and teaming up on therapy designs that address the all encompassing necessities of the patient. The consistent coordination of care inside a solitary foundation disposes of the requirement for patients to explore between numerous offices, smoothing out their medical services venture.

The cooperative model in multispeciality clinics reaches out to interdisciplinary groups that talk about cases, share information, and on the whole add to the patient's prosperity. For instance, a patient with diabetes might profit from the skill of endocrinologists, nutritionists, and actual specialists cooperating to exhaustively deal with the condition. This cooperative methodology lines up with the all encompassing recuperating worldview, perceiving the interaction between various parts of wellbeing.

Patient-Driven Care:

Multispeciality clinics focus on tolerant driven care as a principal part of all encompassing mending. This approach perceives that every patient is a remarkable person with unmistakable necessities, inclinations, and conditions. Patient-focused care includes drawing in patients in shared navigation, regarding their qualities and inclinations, and taking into account the effect of wellbeing mediations on their general personal satisfaction.

In multispeciality clinics, a patient's process is seen thoroughly, considering the particular condition being treated as well as the more extensive setting of their wellbeing. This might imply tending to basic gamble factors, taking into account the patient's psychological and close to home prosperity, and integrating preventive measures into the treatment plan. Patient-driven care is especially significant in constant illness the executives, where continuous coordinated effort among patients and medical services suppliers is fundamental.

Correspondence and shared independent direction are key parts of patient-driven care inside multispeciality medical clinics. Guaranteeing that patients approach data, grasp their treatment choices, and effectively partake in choices about their wellbeing enables them to take responsibility for prosperity. This cooperative methodology cultivates a feeling of trust and organization among patients and medical care suppliers, adding to a good and steady mending climate.

Preventive Measures and Health Projects:

All encompassing mending puts major areas of strength for an on preventive measures to keep up with ideal wellbeing and prosperity. Multispeciality clinics assume a crucial part in preventive consideration by offering wellbeing programs, wellbeing screenings, and instructive drives. These projects plan to distinguish risk factors, recognize potential medical problems early, and enable people to settle on informed way of life decisions that advance long haul wellbeing.

Preventive consideration inside multispeciality medical clinics goes past normal check-ups and screenings. It includes a proactive way to deal with wellbeing advancement, tending to way of life factors like sustenance, actual work, and stress the board. For instance, a multispeciality emergency clinic might offer studios on solid cooking, wellness classes, and stress decrease methods as a feature of its health programs.

The incorporation of preventive measures lines up with the comprehensive model of medical services, perceiving that keeping up with wellbeing isn't exclusively about treating infections yet additionally about encouraging a climate that supports prosperity. By tending to take a chance with factors and advancing sound ways of life, multispeciality emergency clinics add to the counteraction of illnesses and the upgrade of generally speaking personal satisfaction for their patients.

The executives of Ongoing Circumstances:

Constant circumstances, like diabetes, hypertension, and joint pain, frequently require progressing the executives and a diverse way to deal with care. Multispeciality clinics are strategically situated to address the intricate necessities of patients with persistent circumstances by offering thorough and composed types of assistance. The cooperative endeavors of experts from different disciplines add to a comprehensive treatment plan that thinks about both the prompt and long haul parts of the patient's wellbeing.

In the administration of persistent circumstances, multispeciality emergency clinics might consolidate a scope of mediations, including medicine the executives, non-intrusive treatment, dietary directing, and mental help. This exhaustive methodology perceives that ongoing circumstances are much of the time impacted by various variables, including hereditary qualities, way of life, and ecological contemplations.

Moreover, the mix of all encompassing modalities, like needle therapy, yoga, and care rehearses, can supplement customary clinical mediations in the administration of persistent circumstances. These modalities address the actual side effects as well as the psychological and close to home parts of residing with a constant disease. Multispeciality medical clinics, with their different scope of administrations, are appropriate to give these integrative methodologies, adding to the all encompassing prosperity of people with ongoing circumstances.

High level Diagnostics and Innovation:

The job of multispeciality clinics in all encompassing recuperating is altogether upgraded by their admittance to cutting edge diagnostics and innovation. Current medical care depends on modern imaging, research facility tests, and clinical advances to analyze conditions precisely and guide therapy choices. Multispeciality clinics are outfitted with cutting edge offices, taking into consideration a complete evaluation of patients' wellbeing.

High level diagnostics empower medical care suppliers to identify illnesses in their beginning phases, frequently before side effects manifest. This early identification is urgent for opportune mediation and preventive measures. Multispeciality medical clinics, with their coordinated methodology, can guarantee that patients get a brief and exhaustive indicative assessment, considering a more proactive and successful reaction to wellbeing challenges.

Mechanical headways likewise work with correspondence and coordination among medical care groups inside multispeciality clinics. Electronic wellbeing records (EHRs) and computerized correspondence stages smooth out the trading of data, guaranteeing that experts approach a patient's finished clinical history and treatment plan. This consistent progression of data adds to the congruity of care and improves the cooperative endeavors of medical services suppliers.

Far reaching Careful and Clinical Intercessions:

Multispeciality emergency clinics are prepared to give many careful and clinical intercessions, tending to conditions that require specific skill. Whether it's complicated medical procedures, organ transfers, or high level clinical therapies, the accessibility of different experts inside a similar establishment guarantees that patients get thorough and coordinated care.

For instance, a patient with cardiovascular issues might require the skill of cardiologists, cardiothoracic specialists, and vascular specialists. In a multispeciality emergency clinic, these experts can team up to foster a custom fitted therapy plan that envelops clinical administration, interventional methods, and careful mediations. The accessibility of a thorough scope of administrations inside a similar foundation limits defers in treatment and enhances patient results.

Joining of All encompassing Modalities:

Comprehensive mending envelops the acknowledgment that wellbeing is affected by different interconnected factors, including mental, profound, and otherworldly prosperity. Multispeciality medical clinics are progressively integrating comprehensive modalities into their contributions, perceiving the benefit of tending to the entire individual in the mending system.

All encompassing modalities might incorporate integrative treatments, for example, needle therapy, knead, care based pressure decrease, and craftsmanship treatment. These modalities, frequently established in customary recuperating rehearses, add to the general prosperity of patients by tending to viewpoints past the actual side effects of ailment.

Coordinating comprehensive modalities lines up with the standards of patient-focused care and encourages a climate that supports recuperating on various levels.

Difficulties and Valuable open doors:

While multispeciality emergency clinics assume a vital part in comprehensive mending, they face difficulties that warrant consideration for proceeded with progress and development.

Correspondence and Coordination:

The consistent coordination of care among different claims to fame is fundamental for comprehensive mending. In any case, correspondence difficulties can emerge, prompting divided care. Guaranteeing powerful correspondence and interdisciplinary cooperation requires vigorous frameworks, normalized conventions, and a pledge to encouraging a culture of collaboration inside the emergency clinic.

Social Capability:

Multispeciality medical clinics serve assorted patient populaces, each with remarkable social foundations and convictions. Social skill among medical services suppliers is critical for understanding and regarding the different requirements of patients. Preparing projects and drives to advance social mindfulness can add to a more comprehensive and patient-focused way to deal with care.

Preventive Consideration Accentuation:

While preventive consideration is a foundation of all encompassing recuperating, its mix into routine medical services rehearses requires a change in mentality. Empowering medical services suppliers to focus on preventive measures, instruct patients on solid ways of life, and integrate wellbeing programs into routine consideration is a continuous chance for development.

Tending to Emotional well-being:

All encompassing recuperating recognizes the interconnectedness of mental and actual prosperity. Multispeciality medical clinics have a chance to additionally incorporate psychological wellness administrations into their all encompassing consideration models. This includes destigmatizing psychological wellness issues, guaranteeing admittance to emotional well-being experts, and elevating a cooperative way to deal with tending to both mental and actual wellbeing concerns.

Patient Schooling and Strengthening:

Comprehensive mending accentuates patient commitment and strengthening. Multispeciality emergency clinics can improve patient schooling drives, giving assets that engage people to take part in their wellbeing effectively. This incorporates instructive materials, studios, and computerized devices that help patients in settling on informed conclusions about their prosperity.

Incorporation of Innovation:

While cutting edge innovation adds to the indicative capacities of multispeciality medical clinics, improving the incorporation of innovation stays a continuous test. Resolving issues like interoperability, information security, and guaranteeing that innovation upgrades, instead of reduces, the patient-supplier relationship are basic contemplations.

3.1 Comprehensive Patient Care

Far reaching Patient Consideration: Supporting Comprehensive Prosperity in Medical services

Complete patient consideration addresses a worldview in medical services that rises above the ordinary model of treating secluded sicknesses and side effects. It epitomizes an all encompassing methodology that considers the physical, mental, close to home, and social elements of a patient's prosperity. This investigation digs into the standards, parts, and meaning of thorough patient consideration, inspecting how it encourages a more profound comprehension of patients' requirements, improves wellbeing results, and adds to a more humane and patient-focused medical services framework.

Standards of Exhaustive Patient Consideration:

At the center of complete patient consideration are a few core values that shape the conveyance of medical care administrations. These standards stress an all encompassing comprehension of patients as the need might arise, encounters, and settings. Key standards include:

Patient-Centeredness:

Complete patient consideration puts the patient at the focal point of the medical services insight. It perceives the significance of understanding and regarding patients' qualities, inclinations, and objectives. Patient-focused care includes drawing in patients in shared direction, effectively including them in their treatment designs, and taking into account their points of view in the dynamic cycle.

Comprehensive Viewpoint:

An all encompassing viewpoint is essential to exhaustive patient consideration, it is diverse and interconnected to recognize that wellbeing. This point of view goes past the treatment of explicit infections and side effects to consider the more extensive determinants of wellbeing, including way of life factors, social determinants, and the effect of mental and close to home prosperity on actual wellbeing.

Interdisciplinary Joint effort:

Complete patient consideration includes coordinated effort among medical services experts from different disciplines.

Interdisciplinary groups, containing doctors, attendants, subject matter experts, specialists, and other medical services suppliers, cooperate to address the different requirements of patients. This cooperative methodology guarantees that the intricacies of patients' wellbeing are considered according to various viewpoints.

Congruity of Care:

Guaranteeing congruity of care is fundamental to extensive patient consideration. This includes a consistent progress of care across various medical services settings, from essential consideration to specialty care and, if important, to hospitalization and post-release follow-up. Progression of care adds to better coordination, decreased clinical blunders, and worked on persistent results.

Preventive Concentration:

Exhaustive patient consideration puts major areas of strength for an on preventive measures to keep up with ideal wellbeing and prosperity. This incorporates wellbeing screenings, immunizations, way of life guiding, and early intercession to distinguish and address risk factors before they lead to huge medical problems. The preventive center lines up with the more extensive objective of advancing generally wellbeing.

Parts of Far reaching Patient Consideration:

Exhaustive patient consideration involves a scope of parts that on the whole add to tending to the different requirements of people. These parts include the finding and treatment of sicknesses as well as angles connected with psychological wellness, preventive consideration, patient schooling, and emotionally supportive networks. Key parts include:

Extensive Wellbeing Appraisals:

An intensive and exhaustive wellbeing evaluation is the foundation of patient consideration. This includes gathering definite data about a patient's clinical history, current side effects, way of life factors, social determinants, and mental prosperity. Exhaustive wellbeing evaluations give a comprehensive comprehension of the patient's wellbeing status, directing medical services suppliers in fitting mediations to address individual issues.

Coordinated Emotional well-being Administrations:

Psychological wellness is an essential part of exhaustive patient consideration. Incorporated emotional well-being administrations perceive the interconnectedness of mental and actual prosperity. This includes evaluating for emotional well-being issues, giving admittance to psychological well-being experts, and integrating psychological wellness contemplations into the general treatment plan. Addressing psychological wellness adds to a more all encompassing and patient-focused way to deal with care.

Patient Training and Strengthening:

Far reaching patient consideration incorporates vigorous patient schooling drives that enable people to take part in their wellbeing effectively. Patient training includes giving data about ailments, treatment choices, preventive measures, and way of life decisions. Engaged patients are better prepared to come to informed conclusions about their wellbeing, prompting worked on self-administration and adherence to treatment plans.

Preventive Consideration and Wellbeing Advancement:

An emphasis on preventive consideration is vital to thorough patient consideration. This incorporates routine wellbeing screenings, immunizations, way of life directing, and mediations pointed toward decreasing the gamble of infections. Wellbeing advancement drives go past getting sicknesses cultivating a climate that upholds by and large health. Preventive consideration lines up with the standards of thorough patient consideration by tending to wellbeing proactively and taking into account the drawn out prosperity of people.

Cooperative Consideration Groups:

Interdisciplinary and cooperative consideration groups are a vital part of thorough patient consideration. These groups unite medical care experts from different claims to fame to address the assorted requirements of patients by and large. The cooperative model guarantees that patients benefit from the mastery of various medical services suppliers cooperating to foster extensive and facilitated therapy plans.

Social Skill and Variety:

Social skill is pivotal for giving exhaustive patient consideration in assorted social orders. Medical care suppliers should comprehend and regard the social foundations, convictions, and inclinations of patients. This includes fitting consideration intends to oblige social variety, working with viable correspondence, and establishing a comprehensive medical care climate that qualities and regards individual contrasts.

Coordination of Care:

Composed care guarantees that various parts of a patient's treatment plan are flawlessly coordinated. This includes viable correspondence among medical services suppliers, sharing of data, and cooperative independent direction. Coordination reaches out across different medical services settings, guaranteeing that patients experience a smooth continuum of care from essential consideration to specialty care and then some.

Meaning of Extensive Patient Consideration:

The meaning of exhaustive patient consideration is significant, impacting individual wellbeing results as well as the general working of medical services frameworks. A few key viewpoints highlight its significance:

Worked on Quiet Results:

Complete patient consideration adds to further developed wellbeing results by tending to the sum of a patient's wellbeing. This approach perceives that tending to the actual side effects as well as mental, profound, and social elements can prompt more powerful and economical wellbeing enhancements. Further developed results incorporate better administration of constant circumstances, diminished medical clinic readmissions, and improved in general personal satisfaction.

Upgraded Patient Experience:

A patient-focused and thorough way to deal with care improves the general patient experience. Patients feel more drew in, regarded, and engaged with their medical care choices. The accentuation on correspondence, shared direction, and tending to individual requirements encourages a positive and strong medical services climate. Upgraded patient experience adds to more significant levels of patient fulfillment and adherence to treatment plans.

Financially savvy Care:

While extensive patient consideration might include a more proactive and preventive methodology, it can possibly be savvy over the long haul. By tending to medical problems early, forestalling difficulties, and advancing by and large wellbeing, medical services frameworks can decrease the monetary weight related with the therapy of cutting edge or preventable circumstances. Preventive consideration and early mediation can prompt long haul cost investment funds for the two people and medical services frameworks.

Advancement of Populace Wellbeing:

Complete patient consideration lines up with the more extensive objectives of populace wellbeing the executives. By tending to the determinants of wellbeing, advancing preventive measures, and cultivating in general wellbeing, this approach adds to the wellbeing and prosperity of whole populaces. The standards of far reaching patient consideration stretch out past individual patient connections to shape general wellbeing systems and strategies.

Alleviation of Wellbeing Incongruities:

Social capability and a comprehension of social determinants of wellbeing are intrinsic in far reaching patient consideration. This approach perceives the effect of social, monetary, and social elements on wellbeing results. By tending to wellbeing differences and imbalances, extensive patient consideration endeavors to guarantee that medical care administrations are available, comprehensive, and custom-made to the assorted necessities of people and networks.

Long haul Prosperity:

The emphasis on preventive consideration, emotional wellness, and in general health in far reaching patient consideration adds to the drawn out prosperity of people.

It goes past the treatment of intense sicknesses to help people in keeping up with ideal wellbeing and working. This accentuation on long haul prosperity lines up with the developing idea of medical services as a persistent and proactive excursion instead of a receptive reaction to sicknesses.

Challenges in Executing Exhaustive Patient Consideration:

While the standards and parts of complete patient consideration are generally perceived, a few difficulties exist in its viable execution. Tending to these difficulties is essential for understanding the maximum capacity of comprehensive and patient-focused medical care:

Time Imperatives:

Medical services suppliers frequently acknowledgment imperatives in clinical settings, restricting the profundity of cooperations with patients. Complete patient consideration requires intensive evaluations, open correspondence, and cooperative navigation, which might be trying inside the imperatives of time pressures. Tracking down ways of streamlining the utilization of time and focus on tolerant focused connections is fundamental.

Innovative Hindrances:

The rising dependence on electronic wellbeing records (EHRs) and innovation in medical services has the two advantages and difficulties. While innovation can upgrade correspondence and coordination, it additionally presents difficulties connected with information security, interoperability, and the potential for depersonalization in understanding supplier collaborations. Finding some kind of harmony between the upsides of innovation and the human touch is significant.

Labor force Preparing and Instruction:

Extensive patient consideration requires medical services experts to be knowledgeable in interdisciplinary cooperation, social skill, and all encompassing ways to deal with wellbeing. Be that as it may, customary clinical schooling and preparing may not sufficiently get ready medical services suppliers for these perspectives. Tending to holes in schooling and giving continuous preparation open doors are fundamental for cultivating a labor force equipped for conveying exhaustive consideration.

Installment and Repayment Models:

The current installment and repayment models in medical services frequently focus on procedural mediations over far reaching and preventive consideration. Moving towards esteem based care models that boost positive wellbeing results and patient fulfillment is fundamental for adjusting monetary impetuses to the objectives of thorough patient consideration.

Reconciliation of Emotional wellness Administrations:

In spite of developing acknowledgment of the significance of psychological wellness, coordinating emotional well-being administrations into routine medical care stays a test. Shame, restricted admittance to emotional wellness experts, and an absence of normalized conventions for psychological well-being screening obstruct the consistent reconciliation of emotional wellness contemplations into extensive patient consideration.

Wellbeing Data Proficiency:

Patients might confront difficulties in grasping complex wellbeing data, treatment choices, and preventive measures. Wellbeing data education, or the capacity to get to, comprehend, and use wellbeing data, is critical for enabling patients to take part in their consideration effectively. Further developing wellbeing data proficiency requires compelling correspondence techniques and patient instruction drives.

Valuable open doors for Headway:

In spite of difficulties, there are huge open doors for propelling exhaustive patient consideration and further implanting its standards in medical care conveyance:

Innovation as an Empowering agent:

While innovation presents difficulties, it additionally offers chances to upgrade far reaching patient consideration. Telehealth, portable wellbeing applications, and advanced wellbeing stages can work with progressing correspondence among patients and medical services suppliers, support remote observing, and give instruments to patient training. Utilizing innovation as an empowering agent can improve the openness and congruity of care.

Interprofessional Instruction:

Interprofessional instruction programs that unite understudies from different medical services disciplines can encourage a cooperative outlook from the beginning phases of expert turn of events. Setting out open doors for interdisciplinary learning, joint effort, and shared direction can get ready future medical services experts for an extensive way to deal with patient consideration.

Strategy and Installment Changes:

Support for strategy changes and installment changes is fundamental to adjust impetuses to the standards of exhaustive patient consideration. Moving towards esteem based care models, where medical services suppliers are compensated for positive wellbeing results, can energize an emphasis on preventive consideration, patient fulfillment, and generally health.

Local area Commitment:

Drawing in networks in medical services choices and drives is critical for tending to social determinants of wellbeing and decreasing wellbeing variations. Local area based programs, outreach drives, and associations with neighborhood associations can upgrade the effect of thorough patient consideration past the walls of medical care establishments.

Patient Support and Strengthening:

Engaging patients to effectively take part in their consideration requires backing endeavors that advance patient schooling, shared direction, and admittance to wellbeing data. Patient backing associations, computerized wellbeing devices, and local area assets can assume a part in supporting patients in exploring their medical services excursion and pursuing informed decisions.

Exploration and Proof Structure:

Leading exploration on the viability of complete patient consideration models is fundamental for building a strong proof base. This examination can illuminate best practices, guide the improvement of normalized conventions, and show the worth of complete patient consideration in further developing wellbeing results and diminishing medical care costs.

3.2 Collaboration Among Specialties

Cooperation Among Claims to fame: Propelling Medical services Through Interdisciplinary Associations

Cooperation among claims to fame remains as a foundation in the development of present day medical care, rising above customary storehouses to cultivate a more coordinated and patient-focused approach. In the unique scene of clinical science, where the limits between strengths are turning out to be progressively permeable, cooperative endeavors among medical care experts from different fields are fundamental for tending to complex wellbeing challenges. This investigation digs into the importance, advantages, difficulties, and future ramifications of joint effort among strengths, exhibiting how interdisciplinary associations add to progressions in quiet consideration, research, and the general direction of medical care frameworks.

Meaning of Coordinated effort Among Fortes:

The meaning of coordinated effort among fortes lies in its capacity to rise above the limits of a solitary discipline approach and address the diverse idea of wellbeing and sickness. In a time of quickly propelling clinical information and innovation, no single specialty has the expansiveness of mastery expected to comprehend and deal with the complexities of present day medical services thoroughly. The exchange of different variables, including hereditary inclinations, way of life decisions, natural impacts, and social determinants of wellbeing, requires a cooperative and interdisciplinary methodology.

Comprehensive Patient Consideration:

Coordinated effort among fortes empowers a comprehensive way to deal with patient consideration, perceiving that wellbeing is a perplexing transaction of physical, mental, and social elements. At the point when experts from various fields team up, they offer exceptional viewpoints that would be useful, taking into account the particular condition as well as its more extensive ramifications on the patient's general prosperity. This all encompassing methodology adds to more customized and far reaching patient consideration plans.

Enhanced Treatment Plans:

The cooperation of claims to fame upgrades treatment plans, particularly in situations where patients present with various medical problems or conditions influencing different organ frameworks. For example, a patient with diabetes and cardiovascular infection might profit from the planned endeavors of endocrinologists and cardiologists, guaranteeing that treatment systems adjust to address the interrelated parts of these circumstances.

Improved Indicative Precision:

Interdisciplinary coordinated effort upgrades analytic precision by utilizing the aptitude of experts with various demonstrative modalities. Consolidating the bits of knowledge of radiologists, pathologists, and clinical subject matter experts, for instance, can prompt a more exact and nuanced comprehension of perplexing clinical cases. This interdisciplinary demonstrative methodology is especially important in testing and vague clinical situations.

Development and Exploration Progressions:

Cooperation among claims to fame drives development and examination headways by cultivating the cross-fertilization of thoughts and techniques. Interdisciplinary exploration groups unite researchers, clinicians, and specialists from different fields, making a fruitful ground for development. This cooperative exploration approach speeds up the interpretation of logical disclosures into clinical applications and adds to the headway of clinical information.

Productive Asset Usage:

By teaming up, strengths can improve asset usage in medical services settings. Shared offices, hardware, and staff can be all the more proficiently utilized when numerous fortes cooperate. This proficiency is especially pertinent with regards to medical services frameworks confronting asset limitations, where joint effort guarantees that assets are utilized sensibly to help a more extensive range of patients.

Advantages of Cooperation Among Claims to fame:

The advantages of cooperation among claims to fame are diverse, affecting patient results, proficient turn of events, and the general viability of medical services conveyance. These advantages highlight the groundbreaking capability of interdisciplinary associations in reshaping the scene of medical services.

Exhaustive Patient-Focused Care:

Cooperation among claims to fame works with exhaustive patient-focused care by uniting specialists to address the different necessities of people. Patients benefit from a group of medical services experts who work cooperatively to foster customized care designs that think about their particular circumstances as well as their inclinations, values, and more extensive wellbeing setting.

Cross-Disciplinary Skill:

Interdisciplinary joint effort bridles cross-disciplinary mastery, permitting experts to take advantage of the information and abilities of partners from various fields. This aggregate mastery is especially important in complex cases that require a combination of information from different strengths. Cross-disciplinary coordinated effort can prompt creative arrangements and worked on understanding results.

Decreased Discontinuity of Care:

Cooperative endeavors among claims to fame add to the decrease of care fracture, where patients might get separated or duplicative administrations from various medical services suppliers. Through incorporated care groups, experts can impart really, share data, and direction their endeavors, guaranteeing that patients experience a consistent continuum of care across various claims to fame.

Upgraded Correspondence and Coordination:

Compelling correspondence and coordination are inborn advantages of cooperation among fortes. Medical services experts from various disciplines figure out how to communicate in a typical language, share bits of knowledge, and take part in interdisciplinary discoursed. Upgraded correspondence works on the comprehension of every specialty's commitments, prompting more durable and patient-focused care conveyance.

Interprofessional Learning and Development:

Interdisciplinary joint effort cultivates interprofessional learning and development among medical services experts. Teaming up with partners from various strengths gives potential open doors to consistent learning, openness to different points of view, and the improvement of a more all encompassing comprehension of patient consideration. This interprofessional approach adds to the continuous expert advancement of medical care groups.

Streamlined Asset Usage:

Joint effort among strengths upgrades the utilization of assets, decreasing overt repetitiveness and further developing effectiveness in medical care conveyance. Shared offices, hardware, and care staff can be used all the more really when claims to fame work cooperatively. This expands the effect of accessible assets as well as adds to financially savvy and feasible medical care rehearses.

Creative Treatment Modalities:

The cooperative energy created by coordinated effort among claims to fame frequently prompts the improvement of imaginative treatment modalities. For instance, the crossing point of a medical procedure, radiology, and oncology might bring about original ways to deal with disease therapy. These creative modalities, conceived out of interdisciplinary cooperation, can possibly change the scene of restorative intercessions.

Challenges in Coordinated effort Among Fortes:

While coordinated effort among fortes offers significant advantages, it isn't without its difficulties. Beating these difficulties is pivotal for understanding the maximum capacity of interdisciplinary associations and guaranteeing that cooperative endeavors convert into worked on tolerant results.

Correspondence Boundaries:

Correspondence boundaries, remembering contrasts for wording and correspondence styles among claims to fame, can hinder compelling joint effort. Defeating these obstructions requires the improvement of normalized correspondence conventions, interdisciplinary preparation programs, and the development of a cooperative culture that values open correspondence.

Social Contrasts:

Fortes frequently have unmistakable expert societies and standards, which can make difficulties in interdisciplinary cooperation. Beating social contrasts requires a promise to encouraging a common character among medical care experts, stressing shared objectives, and establishing a cooperative climate that commends variety and inclusivity.

Primary and Hierarchical Obstacles:

The authoritative construction of medical services situation, including inflexible progressive systems and departmental storehouses, can present obstacles to coordinated effort among fortes. Beating primary hindrances includes reconsidering hierarchical designs, cultivating a culture of cooperation, and carrying out strategies that boost interdisciplinary collaboration.

Time Requirements:

Medical care experts acknowledgment imperatives in their clinical obligations, which might restrict their capacity to participate in cooperative exercises. Beating time requirements requires focusing on cooperation as a fundamental part of expert work on, giving devoted opportunity to interdisciplinary gatherings, and perceiving and compensating cooperative endeavors.

Extent of-Practice Concerns:

Explaining and exploring extent of-practice concerns is vital in interdisciplinary coordinated effort. Medical care experts should have a reasonable comprehension of their jobs and obligations inside the cooperative group. This requires continuous instruction, normalized conventions, and a common obligation to working inside the limits of every specialty's mastery.

Protection from Change:

Protection from change, whether established in proficient practices or individual inclinations, can represent a huge test to interdisciplinary coordinated effort. Defeating opposition includes proactive initiative, instruction on the advantages of cooperation, and making a culture that values constant improvement and variation to developing medical care standards.

Restricted Interdisciplinary Preparation:

Restricted open doors for interdisciplinary preparation during proficient instruction can obstruct cooperative endeavors. Incorporating interdisciplinary preparation into clinical and medical services instruction programs is fundamental for getting ready people in the future of medical services experts to work flawlessly across claims to fame.

Future Ramifications and Potential open doors:

The future ramifications of coordinated effort among fortes are sweeping, holding the possibility to reshape medical services conveyance, exploration, and training. Perceiving the developing scene, a few open doors and areas of center arise for progressing interdisciplinary joint effort:

Innovation as a Facilitator:

Innovation assumes a urgent part in defeating a portion of the difficulties related with cooperation among strengths. Telehealth stages, electronic wellbeing records (EHRs), and advanced specialized instruments can work with constant data trade, virtual meetings, and interdisciplinary conversations, defeating geological obstructions and upgrading cooperation.

Interdisciplinary Exploration Drives:

What's in store holds energizing possibilities for interdisciplinary examination drives that unite specialists from various fields to address complex medical care difficulties. Cooperative exploration endeavors can prompt historic revelations, inventive medicines, and a more profound comprehension of the interconnected elements impacting wellbeing and infection.

Upgraded Interprofessional Schooling:

Putting resources into improved interprofessional training is basic for planning medical services experts for cooperative practice. Incorporating interdisciplinary preparation modules into clinical and medical services instruction projects can cultivate a culture of coordinated effort from the beginning phases of expert turn of events.

Strategy and Installment Changes:

Pushing for strategy and installment changes that boost and backing interdisciplinary cooperation is fundamental. Moving towards esteem based care models that reward positive wellbeing results and cooperative endeavors can establish a helpful climate for medical services experts to work cooperatively.

Local area Focused Medical care:

Future medical care models may progressively zero in on local area focused approaches, where coordinated effort among claims to fame stretches out past conventional medical services settings. Drawing in networks in medical services choices, utilizing local area assets, and encouraging associations with nearby associations can improve the effect of cooperative endeavors.

Patient-Driven Cooperative Consideration:

The fate of medical care imagines a patient-driven approach where joint effort among strengths is driven by the novel requirements and inclinations of individual patients. Fitting cooperative consideration intends to line up with patient objectives, values, and way of life decisions guarantees that medical services endeavors are really understanding focused and receptive to different necessities.

Worldwide Wellbeing Coordinated efforts:

Coordinated effort among fortes isn't restricted to individual medical services frameworks or locales. Future open doors incorporate worldwide wellbeing joint efforts where specialists from various strengths team up on tending to worldwide wellbeing challenges, sharing information, and adding to the improvement of impartial and available medical services arrangements around the world.

3.3 Holistic Approach to Diagnosis and Treatment

All encompassing Way to deal with Determination and Treatment: Sustaining Complete Medical care

In the steadily developing scene of medical care, a comprehensive way to deal with conclusion and therapy has arisen as a change in perspective, testing customary models that frequently center around secluded side effects or sicknesses. An all encompassing point of view recognizes the interconnectedness of different parts of a singular's wellbeing, perceiving that physical, mental, profound, and social factors on the whole impact prosperity. This investigation digs into the standards, parts, advantages, and difficulties of taking on an all encompassing way to deal with conclusion and treatment, exhibiting how this approach adds to more customized, patient-focused, and powerful medical services.

Standards of Comprehensive Determination and Treatment:

At the core of the comprehensive way to deal with determination and treatment are a few core values that shape how medical services is conceptualized and conveyed. These standards include a wide comprehension of wellbeing and health, underlining the significance of tending to different components of a singular's life.

Acknowledgment of Interconnectedness:

The comprehensive methodology perceives the unpredictable interconnectedness of different parts of wellbeing. It goes past treating separated side effects or infections and considers the transaction between physical, mental, profound, and social elements. This interconnected view recognizes that these aspects are not discrete elements but rather essential parts of an individual's general prosperity.

Individualization of Care:

All encompassing medical services underlines the individualization of care, perceiving that every individual is extraordinary and answers diversely to therapies. Instead of applying normalized conventions, the all encompassing methodology tailors finding and treatment plans to the particular necessities, inclinations, and conditions of the person. This individualized center encourages a more persistent driven and customized way to deal with medical care.

Counteraction and Wellbeing Advancement:

Counteraction is a foundation of the comprehensive methodology, intending to address wellbeing challenges proactively as opposed to responsively treating sicknesses. This includes overseeing existing circumstances as well as advancing health and forestalling the beginning of illnesses. Health advancement systems might incorporate way of life alterations, stress the board, and training on preventive measures.

Thought of Psyche Body Association:

The comprehensive methodology perceives the unpredictable association between the brain and body. Mental and close to home prosperity are viewed as fundamental parts of in general wellbeing. This viewpoint recognizes that mental variables can influence actual wellbeing, as well as the other way around. Treatments and intercessions frequently target both the psychological and actual aspects to accomplish comprehensive prosperity.

Patient Strengthening and Commitment:

Comprehensive medical services puts serious areas of strength for an on understanding strengthening and commitment. Patients are urged to effectively partake in their medical services venture, pursue informed choices, and take responsibility for prosperity. This cooperative methodology between medical care suppliers and patients cultivates a feeling of strengthening and responsibility for one's wellbeing.

Parts of Comprehensive Conclusion and Treatment:

The all encompassing way to deal with determination and treatment contains a scope of parts that on the whole add to a thorough and integrative model of medical care. These parts go past customary clinical evaluations and mediations, enveloping way of life factors, profound prosperity, and the more extensive social setting.

Complete Wellbeing Appraisals:

All encompassing determination starts with thorough wellbeing evaluations that stretch out past the recognizable proof of side effects. These evaluations incorporate an exhaustive survey of clinical history, way of life variables, stressors, and profound prosperity. Professionals might investigate dietary propensities, rest designs, work-out schedules, and natural impacts to acquire a comprehensive comprehension of the singular's wellbeing.

Coordination of Customary and Elective Medication:

The comprehensive methodology frequently coordinates customary clinical practices with option and correlative treatments. This reconciliation perceives that different modalities, including needle therapy, home grown medication, care, and yoga, can add to generally speaking prosperity. The blend of proof based medication and comprehensive treatments gives a more different and adaptable scope of treatment choices.

Nourishing and Way of life Intercessions:

Comprehensive medical services puts huge accentuation on the job of nourishment and way of life in wellbeing and illness. Specialists might recommend dietary changes, nourishing enhancements, and way of life adjustments as a feature of the treatment plan. This all encompassing viewpoint recognizes the effect of way of life factors on wellbeing results and tries to engage people to go with decisions that help prosperity.

Mind-Body Treatments:

The psyche body association is vital to comprehensive medical care, and different brain body treatments are incorporated into therapy plans. Practices like contemplation, biofeedback, directed symbolism, and unwinding strategies plan to advance mental and profound prosperity, ease pressure, and backing the body's normal recuperating processes.

Profound and Mental Help:

All encompassing determination and treatment remember a concentration for close to home and mental prosperity. Psychological well-being appraisals, guiding, and psychotherapeutic intercessions are incorporated into all encompassing consideration plans. Perceiving the effect of pressure, injury, and profound elements on wellbeing, experts endeavor to address these viewpoints to advance all encompassing prosperity.

Social Determinants of Wellbeing Thought:

The comprehensive methodology reaches out past individual elements to think about friendly determinants of wellbeing. This includes perceiving the impact of social, monetary, and natural elements on wellbeing results. Specialists might resolve issues like lodging, business, and admittance to assets, understanding that these variables add to the general wellbeing of people and networks.

Advantages of All encompassing Finding and Treatment:

The reception of an all encompassing way to deal with finding and treatment offers a huge number of advantages that reach out past side effect the board. These benefits add to worked on persistent results, improved prosperity, and a more understanding focused medical services insight.

Worked on Persistent Results:

All encompassing finding and treatment add to worked on quiet results by tending to wellbeing challenges at different levels. The thought of physical, mental, and social aspects permits professionals to foster far reaching care designs that focus on the main drivers of conditions, prompting more reasonable and viable results.

Upgraded Personal satisfaction:

The all encompassing methodology centers around restoring infections as well as on improving the general personal satisfaction. By tending to way of life factors, profound prosperity, and social determinants of wellbeing, people experience enhancements in their everyday working, versatility to stretch, and a feeling of in general prosperity.

Counteraction of Ongoing Circumstances:

Comprehensive medical care puts areas of strength for an on preventive measures, expecting to address risk factors and advance generally speaking health. By proactively tending to way of life factors, offering preventive mediations, and cultivating sound propensities, the comprehensive methodology adds to the avoidance of persistent circumstances and the support of ideal wellbeing.

Patient-Focused Care Insight:

Comprehensive medical services focuses on the singular requirements and inclinations of patients, cultivating a more quiet focused care insight. Patients feel appreciated, regarded, and effectively participated in their medical care choices. This patient-focused approach adds to more significant levels of fulfillment, adherence to treatment plans, and a positive medical services venture.

Strengthening and Taking care of oneself Abilities:

All encompassing medical services enables people to take part in their wellbeing and prosperity effectively. Patients gain information about the interconnected parts of wellbeing, master taking care of oneself abilities, and settle on informed conclusions about their ways of life. This strengthening adds to a feeling of organization and obligation regarding one's wellbeing.

Decrease of Polypharmacy:

The integrative idea of all encompassing medical care frequently brings about a more prudent utilization of drugs. By tending to basic way of life and natural elements, professionals might lessen the dependence on numerous drugs, limiting expected secondary effects and further developing generally medicine the executives.

Comprehensive Way to deal with Constant Circumstances:

Persistent circumstances frequently include complex communications between different elements of wellbeing. All encompassing finding and therapy give a more nuanced and exhaustive way to deal with overseeing ongoing circumstances. By considering the physical, close to home, and social parts of these circumstances, professionals can foster all encompassing techniques that work on long haul results.

Cultivating Versatility and Adapting Abilities:

The accentuation on profound and mental prosperity in all encompassing medical care cultivates the advancement of versatility and adapting abilities. People learn systems to explore pressure, adapt to difficulties, and assemble profound prosperity. This emphasis on strength adds to a more all encompassing and proactive way to deal with psychological well-being.

Challenges in Executing All encompassing Determination and Treatment:

Regardless of its many advantages, the reception of an all encompassing way to deal with determination and treatment faces a few difficulties. These difficulties range from foundational obstructions inside medical services frameworks to social discernments and restrictions in current clinical schooling.

Restricted Joining in Medical care Frameworks:

Customary medical care frameworks might have designs and work processes that are not intrinsically intended to oblige all encompassing methodologies. Restricted combination of all encompassing practices inside standard medical services can obstruct the consistent reception of these methodologies and may bring about divided care.

Social and Expert Obstruction:

Social and expert protection from comprehensive methodologies can introduce a critical test. Some medical care experts, foundations, or people might be impervious to integrating contemporary or corresponding treatments into their training. Tending to these social and expert predispositions is pivotal for the inescapable acknowledgment of all encompassing medical services.

Inadequate Preparation and Schooling:

Medical services experts might get restricted preparing in comprehensive methodologies during their schooling.

The absence of openness to comprehensive standards, integrative medication, and the interconnected idea of wellbeing can thwart the reception of all encompassing practices. Coordinating all encompassing instruction into clinical and medical care preparing programs is fundamental for setting up the up and coming age of medical care suppliers.

Protection and Repayment Difficulties:

The ongoing medical services repayment models frequently favor explicit strategies and therapies instead of comprehensive and preventive methodologies. Protection inclusion and repayment for comprehensive administrations might be restricted, presenting monetary difficulties for both medical services suppliers and patients keen on all encompassing consideration. Promotion for changes in repayment models is essential for the boundless reception of all encompassing methodologies.

Absence of Normalization and Proof:

Comprehensive practices incorporate many treatments, and the absence of normalization can be a test. The shifting levels of proof supporting different comprehensive intercessions might add to incredulity inside the clinical local area. Laying out normalized conventions and leading vigorous exploration on the viability of all encompassing methodologies are fundamental stages in tending to this test.

Coordination among Specialists:

All encompassing medical care frequently includes joint effort among experts from various disciplines, and coordination among these experts can challenge. Laying out successful correspondence channels, interdisciplinary cooperation, and shared dynamic cycles are basic for giving durable and coordinated all encompassing consideration.

Insight and Understanding:

Patient and supplier insights and comprehension of all encompassing medical care can change. A few people might see all encompassing methodologies as eccentric or doubtful, while others might embrace these methodologies as indispensable to their prosperity. Upgrading public mindfulness, instruction, and correspondence about the standards and advantages of all encompassing medical services is urgent for evolving insights.

Open doors for Progression:

Tending to the difficulties related with executing an all encompassing way to deal with conclusion and treatment requires proactive measures and valuable open doors for progression inside the medical services scene.

Coordination into Medical care Arrangements:

Backing for the incorporation of all encompassing standards into medical services approaches is essential.

This incorporates advancing strategies that perceive the worth of comprehensive methodologies, support repayment for all encompassing administrations, and energize the consideration of all encompassing schooling in medical care preparing programs.

Research on Comprehensive Intercessions:

Leading thorough examination on the viability and security of all encompassing intercessions is fundamental for building a proof base. Strong logical examinations can add to the normalization of all encompassing practices, guide clinical independent direction, and improve the validity of comprehensive methodologies inside the clinical local area.

Interdisciplinary Preparation Projects:

Coordinating interdisciplinary preparation programs into clinical and medical services training can overcome any issues in understanding and cooperation among professionals. These projects can open medical care experts to all encompassing standards, energize cooperation between various fortes, and cultivate a more comprehensive and cooperative medical services culture.

Patient Schooling and Promotion:

Enabling patients through training and support is basic for changing insights and cultivating acknowledgment of all encompassing medical care. Patient backing gatherings, instructive drives, and local area commitment endeavors can assume an essential part in expanding mindfulness about all encompassing methodologies and their likely advantages.

Innovation and Telehealth Mix:

Utilizing innovation, including telehealth stages, can improve the availability and reconciliation of all encompassing medical services. Virtual discussions, advanced wellbeing devices, and remote observing can work with all encompassing consideration conveyance, particularly for people in underserved or distant regions.

Joint effort with Customary Medication:

Laying out cooperative systems between comprehensive experts and customary clinical experts can improve the reconciliation of all encompassing methodologies into standard medical care. This joint effort can include shared care plans, interdisciplinary counsels, and common regard for the commitments of the two ways to deal with patient prosperity.

Local area Based Comprehensive Drives:

Local area put together drives that concentration with respect to comprehensive medical services can add to the more extensive acknowledgment of these methodologies. Local area wellbeing programs, health focuses, and associations with neighborhood associations can give assets, support, and all encompassing administrations to different populaces.

Chapter 4

Creating a Healing Environment

Establishing a Recuperating Climate: Sustaining the Prosperity of People

The idea of a recuperating climate rises above the conventional limits of medical services settings, stressing the significance of all encompassing prosperity, solace, and quietness in spaces intended to advance wellbeing and recuperation. This investigation digs into the standards, parts, and advantages of establishing a mending climate, featuring the extraordinary effect it can have on people's physical, close to home, and mental prosperity.

Standards of a Mending Climate:

A mending climate is grounded in major rules that focus on the general prosperity of people inside a given space. These standards include a comprehensive comprehension of wellbeing, perceiving the transaction between actual environmental elements, close to home states, and the recuperating system.

Comprehensive Prosperity:

At the center of a recuperating climate is the affirmation of all encompassing prosperity, which stretches out past the treatment of actual sicknesses. This rule perceives the interconnectedness of physical, mental, and close to home parts of wellbeing. Making a space that takes care of these aspects cultivates a complete way to deal with prosperity.

Solace and Quietness:

A mending climate is portrayed by an emphasis on solace and serenity. This includes contemplations of lighting, temperature, clamor levels, and in general feeling. By developing an environment that advances unwinding and a feeling of safety, people are bound to encounter a good effect on their close to home and mental states.

Patient-Focused Plan:

Patient-focused plan standards are fundamental to establishing a mending climate. This includes fitting actual spaces to address the issues and inclinations of people looking for care. Adaptability in plan, openness, and the consolidation of components that summon a feeling of commonality add to a patient-focused approach.

Association with Nature:

Nature assumes an essential part in a mending climate, with the joining of regular components like daylight, plant life, and perspectives on nature. Openness to nature has been connected to further developed mind-set, diminished feelings of anxiety, and improved generally prosperity. Incorporating biophilic plan standards brings the recuperating force of nature into medical services spaces.

Advancement of Positive Interruptions:

Positive interruptions, like fine art, music, and connecting with visual components, are key parts of a mending climate. These components redirect people's consideration from stressors and add to a more sure close to home insight. Imaginative articulations and tastefully satisfying environmental elements add to a feeling of solace and prosperity.

Parts of a Mending Climate:

Establishing a mending climate includes a smart mix of different parts that on the whole add to a space helpful for prosperity and recuperating. These parts length physical, mental, and tangible perspectives, establishing a climate that supports the brain, body, and soul.

Engineering and Plan:

The structural plan of medical services spaces is a basic part of establishing a recuperating climate. Insightful designs, consolidation of normal light, and the utilization of quieting colors add to an inviting environment. Patient rooms, holding up regions, and normal spaces are planned fully intent on amplifying solace and openness.

Regular Light and Ventilation:

More than adequate normal light and legitimate ventilation are fundamental components in a mending climate. Openness to regular light has been related with further developed state of mind, upgraded rest designs, and a positive effect on circadian rhythms. Satisfactory ventilation adds to a feeling of newness and advances a solid indoor climate.

Workmanship and Style:

Imaginative components, including compositions, models, and different types of innovative articulation, assume a vital part in establishing a recuperating climate. Workmanship has the ability to bring out sure feelings, give a feeling of motivation, and add to an outwardly satisfying climate. Workmanship establishments and feel are cautiously arranged to upgrade the general insight.

Remedial Nurseries and Outside Spaces:

Helpful nurseries and outside spaces are intended to give people open doors for unwinding and association with nature. These spaces might incorporate plant life, strolling ways, and seating regions. Admittance to open air conditions has been displayed to make helpful impacts, advancing pressure decrease and a feeling of quietness.

Innovation Reconciliation:

The reconciliation of innovation is viewed as such that improves instead of cheapens the mending climate. Innovation can be utilized to give amusement, correspondence, and instructive assets. Insightful consolidation of innovation adds to a consistent and patient-accommodating experience.

Agreeable Decorations:

Agreeable decorations, including seating, bedding, and different components, are painstakingly chosen to improve the solace of people in medical services settings. Ergonomic plan standards are applied to guarantee that goods add to a positive and strong experience for patients, guests, and medical care suppliers.

Smell and Tactile Components:

Fragrance based treatment and tactile components add to a multisensory recuperating climate. Lovely fragrances, quieting sounds, and material components are coordinated to make a tangible rich encounter. Fragrance based treatment, specifically, has been connected to unwinding, stress decrease, and positive profound states.

Advantages of Establishing a Recuperating Climate:

The making of a mending climate yields a huge number of advantages that stretch out past actual wellbeing, emphatically influencing people's personal and mental prosperity. These advantages add to a more sure medical care insight and backing the general mending process.

Diminished Pressure and Uneasiness:

A recuperating climate is intended to limit stressors and advance a feeling of serenity. Regular components, relieving colors, and agreeable environmental elements add to a decrease in pressure and tension levels among people looking for care. This decrease in pressure is helpful for the mending system.

Worked on Understanding Fulfillment:

People who experience a recuperating climate frequently report more elevated levels of fulfillment with their medical care encounters. Patient fulfillment is affected by variables like solace, correspondence, and the general vibe of medical services spaces. Positive encounters add to a better impression of medical care administrations.

Improved Profound Prosperity:

Profound prosperity is a focal point of a recuperating climate. The incorporation of workmanship, positive interruptions, and associations with nature decidedly impacts people's personal states. This emphasis on close to home prosperity adds to a more comprehensive and patient-focused way to deal with medical services.

Quicker Recuperation Times:

Studies have recommended that people in mending conditions might encounter quicker recuperation times. The mental and physiological advantages of a positive and strong climate can add to a more proficient recuperating process. Decreased pressure, further developed state of mind, and a feeling of prosperity might add to quicker recuperation directions.

Expanded Staff Fulfillment:

A recuperating climate isn't just useful for patients yet additionally adds to expanded fulfillment among medical care staff. Staff working in conditions that focus on solace, feel, and patient-focused plan might encounter more elevated levels of occupation fulfillment. This, thus, can emphatically affect the nature of care gave.

Support for Family and Guardians:

Recuperating conditions stretch out their positive effect on relatives and guardians. Happy with holding up regions, admittance to outside spaces, and tastefully satisfying environmental factors add to a steady climate for those going with patients. This emotionally supportive network is vital to the general prosperity of people going through medical care encounters.

Advancement of a Positive Medical care Culture:

The formation of recuperating conditions adds to the foundation of a positive medical services culture. Offices that focus on quiet focused plan, all encompassing prosperity, and positive encounters encourage a culture of sympathy, compassion, and a promise to the general prosperity of people.

Challenges in Establishing a Mending Climate:

While the advantages of establishing a mending climate are significant, challenges exist in carrying out and supporting such conditions inside the perplexing scene of medical services. Beating these difficulties requires a deliberate exertion from medical services organizations, creators, and policymakers.

Monetary Limitations:

One of the essential difficulties in establishing recuperating conditions is monetary imperatives. Planning and executing medical care spaces that focus on solace, style, and patient-focused plan might include huge forthright expenses. Offsetting the monetary contemplations with the drawn out benefits requires vital preparation and venture.

Variation to Existing Designs:

Numerous medical care offices are housed in existing designs that may not be helpful for guaranteed changes. Retrofitting existing designs to line up with recuperating climate standards can introduce strategic difficulties. Variation methodologies should be painstakingly considered to limit interruptions while upgrading the recuperating climate.

Normalization versus Customization:

Accomplishing a harmony among normalization and customization represents a test in establishing recuperating conditions. While specific plan components might be normalized for proficiency, customization is pivotal to address the assorted necessities and inclinations of people. Finding some kind of harmony requires smart plan and adaptability in execution.

Protection from Change:

Protection from change inside medical services frameworks, including from staff and overseers, can hinder the reception of recuperating climate standards. Beating obstruction requires powerful correspondence, training, and a common obligation to upgrading the general prosperity of people in medical care settings.

Administrative Consistence:

Medical services offices should stick to administrative principles, which might present difficulties in carrying out specific plan components. Finding some kind of harmony between administrative consistence and the joining of mending climate standards requires cooperation between planners, medical services suppliers, and administrative bodies.

Restricted Mindfulness and Schooling:

Restricted mindfulness and schooling about the advantages of recuperating conditions can block their far and wide reception. Both medical care experts and the overall population may not be completely mindful of the effect of actual environmental elements on wellbeing and prosperity. Training drives are fundamental to advance mindfulness and understanding.

Open doors for Headway:

Propelling the standards of recuperating conditions includes taking advantage of chances for advancement, cooperation, and promotion. These open doors reach out to different partners, including medical care establishments, originators, policymakers, and the more extensive local area.

Examination and Proof Based Plan:

Proceeded with research on the effect of actual conditions on wellbeing results adds to prove based plan. Vigorous logical investigations assist with recognizing the particular components of recuperating conditions that yield positive outcomes. This proof backings the support for integrating recuperating climate standards into medical care rehearses.

Joint effort Among Originators and Medical care Experts:

Joint effort among originators and medical care experts is significant for the fruitful execution of mending conditions. Uniting ability from the two fields guarantees that medical care spaces are stylishly satisfying as well as useful and strong of the general prosperity of people.

Joining of Innovation:

The incorporation of innovation offers chances to upgrade mending conditions. Augmented reality, advanced craftsmanship establishments, and intuitive components can add to positive interruptions and restorative encounters. Innovation can be utilized to establish versatile and dynamic recuperating conditions that answer the different requirements of people.

Local area Commitment and Backing:

Local area commitment and backing drives assume an essential part in propelling recuperating conditions. Drawing in with neighborhood networks, patient backing gatherings, and partners encourages a feeling of shared liability regarding making steady medical services spaces. Promotion endeavors can impact policymakers and drive positive changes in medical care foundation.

Inventive Subsidizing Models:

Investigating imaginative subsidizing models can assist with beating monetary requirements related with establishing mending conditions. Public-private organizations, humanitarian commitments, and awards committed to medical services configuration can give extra assets to carrying out mending climate standards.

Schooling for Medical services Experts:

Schooling programs for medical services experts, including clinicians, managers, and care staff, are fundamental for encouraging a mutual perspective of the significance of mending conditions. Preparing projects can underline the effect of actual spaces on quiet results and the job of medical care experts in establishing steady conditions.

Green Structure and Manageability:

Embracing green structure standards and manageability in medical services configuration lines up with the more extensive objectives of establishing recuperating conditions. Reasonable plan works on, including energy proficiency, utilization of eco-accommodating materials, and incorporation of green spaces, add to both natural maintainability and the prosperity of people.

4.1 Designing Patient-Friendly Spaces

Planning Patient-Accommodating Spaces: A Comprehensive Way to deal with Medical services Conditions

In the domain of medical services, the plan of actual spaces assumes a pivotal part in molding the encounters of patients, parental figures, and medical care experts. Patient-accommodating spaces go past tasteful contemplations, enveloping components that focus on solace, availability, and by and large prosperity. This investigation dives into the standards, parts, difficulties, and valuable open doors in planning patient-accommodating spaces, featuring the groundbreaking effect such conditions can have on the medical services venture.

Standards of Planning Patient-Accommodating Spaces:

Planning patient-accommodating spaces is directed by a bunch of rules that intend to establish conditions helpful for recuperating, solace, and positive encounters. These standards perceive the multi-layered nature of prosperity, underscoring actual well-being as well as the profound and mental parts of the medical care venture.

Patient-Focused Plan:

At the center of planning patient-accommodating spaces is the standard of patient-focused plan. This approach includes effectively thinking about the necessities, inclinations, and encounters of patients in the preparation and design of medical care conditions. It accentuates joint effort between planners, medical services experts, and patients to guarantee that spaces are custom-made to meet individual prerequisites.

Openness and Inclusivity:

Patient-accommodating spaces focus on openness and inclusivity, guaranteeing that conditions are inviting and obliging to people with assorted needs. This incorporates contemplations for people with versatility challenges, visual or hear-able debilitations, and other availability prerequisites. Plan components like inclines, handrails, and clear wayfinding add to a comprehensive climate.

Solace and Serenity:

Solace is a major rule in persistent well disposed plan. From holding up regions to patient rooms, the selection of decorations, lighting, and in general climate is painstakingly considered to establish a calming and agreeable climate. Quietness is incorporated to limit pressure and uneasiness, encouraging a feeling of smoothness helpful for mending.

Adaptability and Versatility:

Patient-accommodating spaces are planned considering adaptability and versatility. The medical care venture is dynamic, and spaces need to oblige assorted exercises and developing requirements. Versatile decorations, particular designs, and multi-functional spaces add to conditions that can be customized to various purposes and phases of care.

Nature and Biophilic Plan:

Integrating components of nature and biophilic plan standards adds to patient-accommodating spaces. Admittance to regular light, perspectives on vegetation, and indoor plants make an association with nature. Biophilic components have been related with pressure decrease, further developed mind-set, and improved in general prosperity.

Parts of Patient-Accommodating Spaces:

Planning patient-accommodating spaces includes an insightful incorporation of different parts that all in all add to conditions advancing prosperity and positive encounters. These parts length structural contemplations, inside plan components, and the general format of medical care offices.

Structural Format:

The structural format of medical care offices frames the groundwork of patient-accommodating plan. Insightful arranging includes contemplations like the situation of patient rooms, holding up regions, and shared spaces. The design ought to work with simple route, limit blockage, and make an intelligent stream that upgrades the general patient experience.

Inviting Meeting rooms:

The meeting room is much of the time the primary resource for patients, and its plan establishes the vibe for the whole medical care insight. Inviting meeting rooms consolidate open to seating, clear signage, and stylishly satisfying plan components. These spaces expect to lessen uneasiness and make a positive initial feeling.

Agreeable Patient Rooms:

Patient rooms are vital to the medical care insight, and their plan is a basic part of patient-accommodating spaces. Happy with bedding, movable lighting, and decorations that make a plain air add to a positive patient encounter. Sufficient protection and spaces for individual possessions further upgrade the solace of patient rooms.

Mitigating Varieties and Lighting:

The selection of varieties and lighting fundamentally influences the air of medical services spaces. Patient-accommodating plan consolidates alleviating colors that advance unwinding and prosperity. Regular lighting is focused on whenever the situation allows, and counterfeit lighting is painstakingly aligned to establish an agreeable and outwardly engaging climate.

Craftsmanship and Style:

Creative components are incorporated into patient-accommodating spaces to improve feel and add to a good environment. Nicely organized fine art, paintings, and models can act as sure interruptions, giving visual interest and making a feeling of association with the more extensive local area.

Wayfinding and Signage:

Compelling wayfinding is pivotal for patient-accommodating spaces, guaranteeing that people can explore medical care offices without any problem. Clear signage, natural wayfinding frameworks, and viewable prompts add to a peaceful encounter for patients and guests. Wayfinding configuration reaches out past directional signage to incorporate visual milestones and reference focuses.

Happy with Holding up Regions:

Holding up regions are spaces where patients and their families invest critical energy. Planning happy with holding up regions includes giving adequate seating, admittance to understanding materials, and contemplations for protection. Making zones inside holding up regions, like calm corners and play regions for kids, adds to a more custom-made insight.

Family and Parental figure Spaces:

Patient-accommodating plan perceives the significance of spaces for relatives and parental figures. Assigned family regions, meeting spaces, and facilities for short term visits are coordinated to help the requirements of those going with patients. These spaces add to a strong climate for the more extensive consideration organization.

Advantages of Patient-Accommodating Plan:

The execution of patient-accommodating plan standards yields a scope of advantages that stretch out to patients, medical care suppliers, and the general medical services framework. These advantages add to worked on persistent results, improved fulfillment, and a more certain medical services insight.

Worked on Quiet Fulfillment:

Patient-accommodating plan essentially adds to worked on persistent fulfillment. Agreeable, stylishly satisfying conditions that focus on individual necessities and inclinations make a positive impression. Positive encounters in medical care spaces are firmly connected to in general fulfillment with medical care administrations.

Decreased Pressure and Uneasiness:

Conditions planned considering the prosperity of patients add to decreased pressure and tension levels. Patient-accommodating spaces consolidate components that advance unwinding, like mitigating tones, agreeable decorations, and admittance to normal light. These plan highlights make a seriously quieting air, emphatically affecting the profound experience of people in medical services settings.

Improved Recuperating Climate:

Patient-accommodating plan adds to the making of recuperating conditions. Agreeable patient rooms, nature-propelled plan components, and positive interruptions on the whole encourage a climate helpful for recuperation. The all encompassing way to deal with patient-accommodating plan perceives the interconnected idea of physical and profound prosperity, supporting the general mending process.

Positive Effect on Staff:

Patient-accommodating plan isn't restricted to helping patients alone; it likewise decidedly influences medical services experts. Agreeable and very much planned work areas add to expanded work fulfillment among medical services staff. A positive work space can upgrade correspondence, cooperation, and generally work execution.

Effective Medical services Conveyance:

All around planned medical services spaces add to more productive medical care conveyance. Smoothed out designs, successful wayfinding, and versatile spaces improve the work process for medical services suppliers. Patient-accommodating plan standards intend to limit clog, diminish stand by times, and improve the general effectiveness of medical care administrations.

Advancement of Preventive Consideration:

Patient-accommodating plan can assume a part in advancing preventive consideration. Agreeable and welcoming medical care conditions might urge people to look for normal check-ups, screenings, and preventive administrations. A positive medical care experience adds to a proactive way to deal with individual prosperity.

Local area Commitment and Trust:

Patient-accommodating spaces add to local area commitment and cultivate trust in medical services organizations. At the point when people see medical care spaces as inviting, open, and receptive to their requirements, there is a more noteworthy probability of local area individuals effectively captivating with medical services administrations. Trust in medical services establishments is fundamental for continuous wellbeing the executives and preventive consideration.

Challenges in Planning Patient-Accommodating Spaces:

Regardless of the clear advantages, planning patient-accommodating spaces isn't without its difficulties. Conquering these difficulties requires a multidisciplinary approach, including joint effort among draftsmen, medical care experts, managers, and patients.

Monetary Requirements:

One of the essential difficulties in planning patient-accommodating spaces is monetary requirements. Carrying out plan components that focus on understanding solace and prosperity might include forthright costs that medical services foundations see as trying to designate.

Offsetting financial plan contemplations with the drawn out advantages of patient-accommodating plan requires key preparation and imaginative subsidizing arrangements.

Adherence to Administrative Norms:

Medical services offices should stick to administrative principles, and these guidelines might impact the plan decisions made in medical services spaces. While principles are fundamental for wellbeing and nature of care, unbending adherence without adaptability can present difficulties in making spaces that are both consistent and patient-accommodating. Finding some kind of harmony requires joint effort between architects, medical care experts, and administrative bodies.

Transformation to Existing Foundation:

Numerous medical services offices work inside existing foundation, which might present difficulties in carrying out quiet agreeable plan components. Retrofitting existing designs to line up with present day plan standards can be strategically perplexing and may require intelligent fixes to adjust without compromising usefulness.

Maintainability Contemplations:

Consolidating feasible plan rehearses while guaranteeing patient-accommodating spaces can challenge. Manageable materials, energy-proficient frameworks, and eco-accommodating drives might have forthright costs that require cautious thought. Offsetting supportability objectives with the prompt requirements of patients includes key preparation and a pledge to long haul natural obligation.

Social Awareness and Variety:

Patient-accommodating plan should be socially touchy and comprehensive of different populaces. Social contrasts, language hindrances, and shifting medical services assumptions might introduce difficulties in making all around quiet accommodating spaces. A thorough comprehension of the social variety inside the patient populace is pivotal for planning spaces that address the issues of everybody.

Valuable open doors for Headway:

Propelling patient-accommodating plan includes jumping all over chances for development, examination, and joint effort. These amazing open doors reach out to planners, medical services foundations, policymakers, and the more extensive local area.

Research on the Effect of Plan:

Proceeded with research on the effect of plan components on understanding results is fundamental for propelling patient-accommodating spaces. Logical investigations can give proof based bits of knowledge into the particular plan includes that add to worked on prosperity, decreased pressure, and positive medical services encounters.

Interdisciplinary Cooperation:

Interdisciplinary joint effort between planners, medical services experts, and scientists is vital to propelling patient-accommodating plan. Uniting skill from different fields guarantees an all encompassing methodology that considers both the tasteful and utilitarian parts of medical services spaces. Cooperative endeavors can prompt creative arrangements and best practices in quiet cordial plan.

Inventive Financing Models:

Investigating inventive subsidizing models can assist with conquering monetary requirements related with patient-accommodating plan. Public-private organizations, altruistic commitments, and awards devoted to medical services configuration can give extra assets to executing plan components that focus on understanding solace and prosperity.

Patient and Local area Commitment:

Effectively including patients and the local area in the plan cycle is a valuable chance to guarantee that patient-accommodating spaces line up with the requirements and assumptions for those they serve. Patient criticism, center gatherings, and local area commitment drives add to a more comprehensive and responsive way to deal with medical care plan.

Instruction for Creators and Medical care Experts:

Instruction programs for originators and medical care experts are fundamental for cultivating a mutual perspective of patient-accommodating plan standards. Preparing projects can stress the effect of actual spaces on understanding encounters and results. Moreover, cross-disciplinary training can improve cooperation among architects and medical services experts.

Support for Patient-Accommodating Plan:

Support endeavors at the institutional and strategy levels can add to the prioritization of patient-accommodating plan. Supporters can attempt to bring issues to light about the advantages of all around planned medical services spaces, impact medical care arrangements, and advance the reconciliation of patient-accommodating plan standards into the preparation and development of new offices.

4.2 Integrating Alternative Therapies

Coordinating Elective Treatments: A Comprehensive Way to deal with Medical care

The scene of medical services is developing, with a rising acknowledgment of the corresponding advantages that elective treatments offer close by traditional clinical therapies. Integrative medication, which consolidates standard clinical treatments with correlative and elective methodologies, has acquired conspicuousness in giving a more all encompassing and patient-focused way to deal with medical services. This investigation dives into the standards, advantages, difficulties, and open doors related with coordinating elective treatments inside the more extensive medical services system.

Standards of Integrative Medication:

Integrative medication is grounded in a few key rules that guide the consolidation of elective treatments into traditional medical care. These standards underscore an all encompassing comprehension of wellbeing, customized treatment plans, and coordinated effort among medical care professionals and patients.

Comprehensive Way to deal with Wellbeing:

At the center of integrative medication is a comprehensive way to deal with wellbeing that perceives the interconnected idea of the body, brain, and soul. As opposed to zeroing in exclusively on the treatment of explicit side effects or sicknesses, integrative medication considers the more extensive elements that add to by and large prosperity, including way of life, nourishment, and profound wellbeing.

Patient-Focused Care:

Integrative medication puts areas of strength for an on persistent focused care, including patients in the dynamic cycle and fitting treatment intends to address individual issues and inclinations. This cooperative methodology encourages an organization between medical care suppliers and patients, enabling people to effectively partake in their medical services venture.

Mix of Ordinary and Elective Treatments:

Integrative medication looks to join the qualities of ordinary clinical medicines with proof based elective treatments. This incorporation depends on an exhaustive comprehension of the logical premise and security of elective methodologies, guaranteeing that they supplement and improve the general viability of regular consideration.

Advancement of Preventive Medication:

Integrative medication puts a huge accentuation on preventive measures and way of life changes to keep up with and further develop wellbeing. By tending to gamble with factors, advancing solid propensities, and offering preventive intercessions, integrative medication adds to the anticipation of constant circumstances and the enhancement of generally prosperity.

Advantages of Coordinating Elective Treatments:

The coordination of elective treatments into medical services gives a scope of advantages that add to a more exhaustive and patient-focused way to deal with prosperity. These advantages range physical, close to home, and mental aspects, tending to the assorted necessities of people looking for medical care.

Improved Treatment Adequacy:

Incorporating elective treatments with traditional clinical medicines can upgrade generally treatment adequacy. A few elective treatments have shown constructive outcomes in overseeing torment, lessening pressure, and working on personal satisfaction.

When joined with regular medicines, this integrative methodology might bring about improved results for specific circumstances.

Further developed Side effect The board:

Elective treatments, like needle therapy, back rub, and care based rehearses, have been displayed to really oversee side effects related with different ailments. Incorporating these treatments into treatment plans can offer people extra instruments for side effect alleviation, particularly for conditions where traditional medicines might have constraints.

Customized and Comprehensive Consideration:

Integrative medication embraces a customized and all encompassing way to deal with care, perceiving that every individual is interesting and may answer distinctively to different helpful modalities. By fitting treatment plans to individual requirements and tending to various elements of wellbeing, integrative medication gives a more exhaustive and patient-focused model of care.

Decreased Results of Customary Medicines:

A few elective treatments, for example, mind-body practices and natural enhancements, may assist with moderating the results of traditional clinical medicines.

Coordinating these treatments can add to a more adjusted and decent medical services insight, working on the general personal satisfaction for people going through clinical mediations.

Strengthening of Patients:

Integrative medication enables patients to play a functioning job in their wellbeing and prosperity. By offering a scope of restorative choices and including patients in navigation, people gain a feeling of organization and responsibility for medical services venture. This strengthening adds to a more sure and drawn in persistent experience.

Upgraded Close to home Prosperity:

Elective treatments that attention on the brain body association, like contemplation and yoga, have been related with enhancements in profound prosperity. Coordinating these practices into medical services can uphold people in adapting to pressure, tension, and personal difficulties, encouraging a more all encompassing way to deal with emotional wellness.

Worked on Personal satisfaction:

The coordination of elective treatments is frequently pointed toward working on the general personal satisfaction for people confronting wellbeing challenges. By tending to actual side effects, profound prosperity, and way of life factors, integrative medication adds to a more comprehensive and positive experience, upgrading the general personal satisfaction for patients.

Challenges in Coordinating Elective Treatments:

While the advantages of coordinating elective treatments are clear, challenges exist in consistently integrating these methodologies into standard medical care. These provokes range from social insights to commonsense contemplations inside medical care frameworks.

Social and Expert Opposition:

Social and expert protection from elective treatments can represent a huge test. A few medical care experts and establishments might be suspicious or reluctant to embrace moves toward that fall outside the customary clinical worldview. Defeating these social and expert predispositions requires training, cooperation, and liberality.

Restricted Exploration and Normalization:

The restricted examination on a few elective treatments and the absence of normalization in practices can be a test in coordinating these methodologies into standard medical care. Laying out strong logical proof, normalized conventions, and rules for the protected and powerful utilization of elective treatments are urgent moves toward tending to this test.

Protection Inclusion and Repayment:

The ongoing medical services repayment models frequently favor explicit operations and drug mediations, leaving restricted inclusion for elective treatments. The absence of protection inclusion and repayment for these treatments can be a boundary for people looking for integrative consideration. Support endeavors are expected to address strategy hindrances and elevate impartial admittance to a scope of restorative choices.

Interdisciplinary Coordinated effort:

Viable mix of elective treatments requires interdisciplinary cooperation among medical services experts from various strengths. Cooperative correspondence and a common perspective of the expected advantages and impediments of elective treatments are fundamental. Conquering storehouses and cultivating coordinated effort can upgrade the consistent mix of these treatments into patient consideration.

Instruction and Preparing:

Both medical care suppliers and the overall population might need sufficient training and mindfulness about elective treatments. Medical care experts might require extra preparation to figure out the standards and uses of different elective methodologies. Patient training is likewise vital to guarantee informed direction and dynamic cooperation in integrative consideration.

Administrative and Permitting Issues:

Administrative structures and permitting guidelines for elective treatments fluctuate generally. Laying out clear guidelines, permitting necessities, and principles for professionals in the field of elective treatments are fundamental to guarantee patient security and nature of care. This requires joint effort between administrative bodies and experts in the field.

Mix into Electronic Wellbeing Records (EHR):

The mix of elective treatments into electronic wellbeing records (EHR) represents a specialized test. Current EHR frameworks are fundamentally intended to catch regular clinical information, and adjusting them to remember data for elective treatments might require updates and alterations. Guaranteeing a consistent progression of data across medical services modalities is basic for giving thorough and composed care.

Potential open doors for Progression:

Propelling the incorporation of elective treatments into standard medical care includes taking advantage of chances for research, instruction, strategy backing, and innovation combination. These valuable open doors reach out to medical services foundations, experts, analysts, and policymakers.

Examination and Proof Based Practices:

Proceeded with research on the security and viability of elective treatments is vital for propelling their mix into standard medical care. Thorough logical examinations add to confirm based works on, laying out an establishment for the consideration of elective treatments in treatment rules and conventions.

Training for Medical care Experts:

Exhaustive training programs for medical care experts, including doctors, nurture, and unified wellbeing suppliers, are fundamental for encouraging a more profound comprehension of elective treatments. Coordinating training on elective methodologies into clinical educational programs and offering proceeding with instruction open doors can improve the information and abilities of medical care experts.

Patient Schooling and Informed Independent direction:
Enabling patients with data about elective treatments is fundamental for informed independent direction. Patient instruction drives can give assets, direction, and clear correspondence about the expected advantages and dangers of elective methodologies. Informed patients are bound to take part in their medical care choices effectively.

Strategy Backing and Repayment Change:
Support endeavors at the strategy level are critical for transforming repayment models and elevating fair admittance to elective treatments. Cooperative drives including medical services experts, patient promotion gatherings, and policymakers can add to strategy changes that help integrative consideration and guarantee fair repayment for elective treatments.

Interdisciplinary Preparation and Cooperation:
Advancing interdisciplinary preparation and cooperation among medical services experts encourages a more all encompassing and cooperative way to deal with patient consideration. Preparing programs that unite professionals from various fortes can upgrade correspondence, understanding, and coordinated effort in giving integrative consideration.

Innovation Mix and EHR Updates:
Progressions in innovation, including updates to electronic wellbeing record (EHR) frameworks, can work with the reconciliation of elective treatments into standard medical care. EHR frameworks ought to be intended to catch significant data about elective methodologies, guaranteeing a complete and composed record of patient consideration.

Local area Based Projects and Focuses:
Laying out local area based integrative medical care projects and focuses can give a strong climate to people looking for elective treatments. These projects can act as center points for schooling, research, and the conveyance of integrative consideration, advancing local area commitment and openness.

4.3 Promoting Mental Well-being in Hospital Settings

Advancing Mental Prosperity in Clinic Settings: An All encompassing Way to deal with Patient Consideration

The meaning of mental prosperity in medical services settings is progressively perceived as a fundamental part of generally speaking patient consideration. Clinics, customarily centered around treating actual illnesses, are developing to embrace a more all encompassing methodology that recognizes the interconnectedness of mental and actual wellbeing. This investigation dives into the standards, difficulties, and methodologies associated with advancing mental prosperity inside the complicated climate of clinic settings.

Standards of Mental Prosperity in Emergency clinics:
Advancing mental prosperity in emergency clinics is grounded in a few key rules that focus on the emotional wellness of patients, families, and medical care experts.

These standards guide the improvement of strategies, practices, and conditions that add to a strong and remedial air.

All encompassing Patient-Focused Care:

At the center of advancing mental prosperity is a guarantee to comprehensive, patient-focused care. Perceiving patients as people with extraordinary psychosocial needs, medical clinics endeavor to incorporate psychological wellness contemplations into generally speaking consideration plans. This includes tending to profound, social, and mental elements that might influence a patient's prosperity.

Nobility and Regard:

Clinics accentuate the significance of treating people with pride and regard, encouraging a climate where patients feel esteemed and heard. This rule reaches out to the language utilized, how data is conveyed, and the general disposition of medical care experts and staff. A culture of regard adds to a positive and steady emotional wellness climate.

Shame Decrease and Instruction:

Clinics take part in endeavors to lessen shame related with emotional well-being conditions. Schooling drives intend to build mindfulness and comprehension of emotional well-being issues among both medical services experts and the more extensive local area. By cultivating sympathy and dispersing legends, emergency clinics add to a climate that empowers open discussions about mental prosperity.

Cooperative Consideration Groups:

The coordination of emotional well-being experts into multidisciplinary care groups is a crucial rule. Cooperative consideration models include coordination among clinical and emotional wellness experts to address both physical and mental parts of patient consideration. This group based approach perceives the interconnected idea of mental and actual wellbeing.

Patient and Family Contribution:

Advancing mental prosperity includes effectively including patients and their families in the consideration cycle. Clinics empower open correspondence, give assets to emotional wellness support, and take part in shared decision-production with patients. By remembering families for conversations and care arranging, medical clinics perceive the more extensive encouraging group of people that adds to mental prosperity.

Challenges in Advancing Mental Prosperity in Emergency clinics:

While the standards of mental prosperity are central, emergency clinics face different difficulties in carrying out viable procedures. Defeating these difficulties requires a thorough and versatile way to deal with address the different necessities of patients and the intricacies of the emergency clinic climate.

Restricted Assets and Financing:

Emergency clinics frequently face asset imperatives and monetary difficulties, which can influence the accessibility of emotional wellness administrations. The designation of adequate assets to help emotional well-being drives, including staffing, preparing, and remedial mediations, is fundamental. Imaginative financing models and backing for emotional wellness subsidizing can assist with tending to this test.

Shame and Attitudinal Boundaries:

Shame encompassing psychological wellness stays a huge obstruction. Attitudinal difficulties among medical care experts, patients, and the more extensive local area can block endeavors to advance mental prosperity. Complete schooling efforts, hostile to shame drives, and social ability preparing are urgent for conquering these hindrances.

Staff Burnout and Prosperity:

Medical services experts, including specialists, attendants, and care staff, may encounter elevated degrees of stress and burnout. The requesting idea of clinic work, particularly in high-pressure conditions, can adversely affect the psychological prosperity of medical care suppliers. Emergency clinics should focus on the prosperity of their staff through help programs, psychological well-being assets, and cultivating a culture of taking care of oneself.

Coordination of Emotional well-being into Essential Consideration:

Coordinating emotional well-being contemplations into essential consideration settings inside emergency clinics represents a test. Complete screenings, convenient references, and the consistent joint effort among clinical and emotional well-being experts are fundamental. Conquering storehouses and encouraging correspondence between various divisions inside a clinic is pivotal for a coordinated way to deal with mental prosperity.

Patient Security and Privacy:

Keeping up with patient security and privacy is a basic thought in emotional wellness care. Emergency clinics should explore the fragile harmony between giving fundamental data to convey exhaustive consideration and regarding the security freedoms of patients. Clear arrangements, moral rules, and staff preparing add to tending to this test.

Crisis and Emergency The board:

Clinics oftentimes experience people in emergency or encountering psychological well-being crises. Really dealing with these circumstances requires specific preparation for medical care experts and a very much organized reaction framework. Clinics need to foster conventions and assets to address emotional wellness emergencies in an ideal and steady way.

Techniques for Advancing Mental Prosperity in Medical clinics:

Tending to the difficulties illustrated above includes the execution of designated techniques that cultivate a culture of mental prosperity inside medical clinics. These systems incorporate a scope of drives, from labor force improvement to natural changes, pointed toward establishing a strong and remedial medical care climate.

Labor force Preparing and Backing Projects:

Extensive preparation programs for medical services experts are fundamental for improving comprehension they might interpret psychological well-being issues and building abilities in tolerant correspondence.

Moreover, emergency clinics can carry out help programs, for example, advising administrations and friend encouraging groups of people, to address the psychological prosperity of their staff.

Incorporated Care Models:

Taking on coordinated care models that flawlessly integrate emotional well-being contemplations into essential consideration is a key system. This includes the co-operation of clinical and emotional wellness experts in the improvement of treatment plans and the arrangement of composed care. The combination of social well-being administrations inside essential consideration settings improves openness and decreases shame.

Local area Organizations and Effort:

Clinics can lay out organizations with local area emotional wellness associations and backing administrations to make a continuum of care. Cooperative endeavors add to a more comprehensive methodology, permitting clinics to interface patients with continuous psychological wellness support upon release. Local area effort and schooling drives likewise assume a part in decreasing shame and advancing emotional wellness mindfulness.

Patient and Family Commitment Projects:

Emergency clinics can execute programs that effectively connect with patients and their families in psychological well-being conversations and care arranging. Giving assets, support gatherings, and instructive materials adds to a cooperative way to deal with mental prosperity. Establishing an inviting climate that empowers open correspondence encourages trust and commitment.

Natural Adjustments:

Clinic conditions can altogether affect mental prosperity. Basic changes, for example, integrating regular light, making quieting spaces, and guaranteeing agreeable facilities, add to a more remedial air. Workmanship establishments, calming variety plans, and green spaces inside emergency clinics can emphatically impact the psychological condition of patients and staff.

Telehealth Administrations for Emotional well-being Backing:

The extension of telehealth administrations offers chances to improve psychological well-being support, particularly in situations where in-person visits might challenge. Telepsychiatry, virtual advising, and remote help administrations empower people to get to psychological wellness care advantageously, diminishing hindrances to looking for help.

Routine Emotional well-being Screenings:

Carrying out routine emotional wellness screenings as a component of standard medical services evaluations distinguishes psychological well-being concerns right off the bat. Ordinary screenings add to a proactive way to deal with mental prosperity, empowering opportune intercessions and backing. Screening instruments can be coordinated into routine clinical visits across different clinic divisions.

Emergency Mediation Preparing for Staff:

Giving emergency mediation preparing to medical care staff outfits them with the abilities to successfully oversee psychological wellness crises. This incorporates de-acceleration methods, correspondence procedures, and coordination with particular emotional well-being emergency groups. Readiness for emergency circumstances adds to a more secure and more steady medical clinic climate.

Chapter 5

Holistic Healing Practices in Multispeciality Hospitals

The scene of medical care is going through an extraordinary shift, with a rising acknowledgment of the significance of all encompassing recuperating rehearses in multispeciality emergency clinics. The expression "comprehensive recuperating" envelops an integrative methodology that addresses the physical, mental, profound, and otherworldly elements of a singular's prosperity. With regards to multispeciality emergency clinics, the consolidation of all encompassing recuperating rehearses connotes a promise to giving thorough and patient-focused care that reaches out past the conventional clinical model. This investigation digs into the standards, advantages, difficulties, and execution procedures related with the mix of comprehensive mending rehearses in the powerful climate of multispeciality clinics.

Standards of Comprehensive Recuperating in Multispeciality Emergency clinics:

Comprehensive recuperating in multispeciality emergency clinics is directed by fundamental rules that focus on the interconnected idea of physical, mental, and close to home wellbeing. These standards shape the ethos of patient consideration, encouraging a climate that recognizes the extraordinary necessities of people and looks to improve their general prosperity.

Entire Individual Methodology:

Comprehensive mending rehearses in multispeciality emergency clinics embrace an entire individual methodology, perceiving that wellbeing reaches out past the shortfall of sickness. This approach considers the physical, mental, close to home, and otherworldly components of an individual, planning to address the main drivers of wellbeing challenges and advance exhaustive prosperity.

Patient-Focused Care:

Fundamental to all encompassing mending in multispeciality emergency clinics is the rule of patient-focused care. This includes effectively including patients in their consideration, taking into account their inclinations, values, and objectives. Emergency clinics endeavor to make associations with patients, cultivating open correspondence and shared decision-production to fit treatment plans to individual necessities.

Incorporation of Corresponding Treatments:

All encompassing mending rehearses frequently include the reconciliation of corresponding treatments close by ordinary clinical medicines. These treatments might incorporate needle therapy, knead, care rehearses, and healthful help. The objective is to offer a range of remedial choices that address the different necessities of patients and improve the general viability of medical services intercessions.

Accentuation on Avoidance and Wellbeing:

All encompassing recuperating in multispeciality medical clinics puts a critical accentuation on preventive measures and health advancement. Past treating intense ailments, clinics participate in proactive wellbeing the board, empowering way of life alterations, wellbeing schooling, and preventive screenings to help people in keeping up with ideal wellbeing.

Social Ability and Variety:

Comprehensive recuperating rehearses focus on social capability and inclusivity. Multispeciality emergency clinics perceive the different foundations, convictions, and upsides of their patient populaces. Socially delicate consideration guarantees that all encompassing mending rehearses are open and aware of the person's social setting.

Advantages of Comprehensive Mending Practices in Multispeciality Clinics:

The fuse of all encompassing mending rehearses in multispeciality emergency clinics yields a huge number of advantages that reach out to patients, medical care suppliers, and the medical services framework overall. These advantages add to worked on persistent results, improved fulfillment, and a more thorough way to deal with medical care conveyance.

Improved Patient Prosperity:

All encompassing mending rehearses add to the general prosperity of patients by tending to their ailments as well as their psychological, profound, and otherworldly requirements. This thorough methodology cultivates a feeling of completeness, emphatically influencing the patient's personal satisfaction and recuperation experience.

Further developed Patient-Supplier Connections:

The patient-focused focal point of comprehensive mending rehearses reinforces the patient-supplier relationship. Open correspondence, shared navigation, and a co-operative way to deal with care add to a feeling of trust and organization among patients and medical services suppliers. This, thus, upgrades the viability of medical care intercessions.

Decrease in Pressure and Nervousness:

Comprehensive recuperating works on, including care based intercessions, back rub, and unwinding methods, add to the decrease of pressure and nervousness levels among patients. These practices establish a helpful climate that upholds close to home prosperity, which is especially useful for people going through clinical medicines.

Extensive Torment The board:

Integrative ways to deal with torment the board, for example, needle therapy, chiropractic care, and brain body procedures, offer extra devices for tending to torment past ordinary clinical medicines. All encompassing recuperating rehearses add to a more far reaching and customized torment the executives technique, limiting the dependence on drugs alone.

Support for Constant Illness The executives:

People with ongoing circumstances frequently benefit from all encompassing recuperating rehearses that accentuate way of life changes, stress decrease, and in general prosperity. Integrative treatments can supplement regular therapies for constant infections, adding to better illness the executives and a superior personal satisfaction.

Positive Effect on Medical services Experts:

The reconciliation of comprehensive mending rehearses decidedly influences medical services experts by cultivating a really satisfying and patient-focused way to deal with care. Suppliers might encounter expanded work fulfillment, decreased burnout, and a feeling of arrangement with the clinic's obligation to all encompassing prosperity.

Improved Patient Fulfillment:

All encompassing mending rehearses add to more elevated levels of patient fulfillment. The customized and exhaustive consideration approach, combined with an emphasis on persistent inclinations and solace, makes a positive medical services insight. Further developed fulfillment is related with better adherence to treatment designs and expanded commitment in medical care.

Challenges in Executing Comprehensive Recuperating Practices:

Regardless of the clear advantages, the coordination of comprehensive recuperating rehearses in multispeciality medical clinics isn't without challenges. Conquering these difficulties requires a key and cooperative methodology including medical care suppliers, overseers, and patients.

Social Shift inside Medical care Frameworks:

Carrying out all encompassing recuperating rehearses frequently requires a social shift inside medical services frameworks. This includes changing dug in standards and perspectives towards medical services conveyance. Protection from change, distrust among some medical services experts, and the requirement for extensive preparation present difficulties in cultivating a comprehensive consideration culture.

Asset Portion and Financing:

The combination of comprehensive mending practices might require extra assets and financing. Complete preparation programs, the work of experts in corresponding treatments, and the production of committed spaces for these practices might bring about forthright expenses. Getting assets and exhibiting the expense adequacy of all encompassing methodologies are difficulties in numerous medical services settings.

Normalization and Proof Based Practices:

Normalizing all encompassing mending rehearses and guaranteeing their arrangement with proof based approaches can challenge. The field of reciprocal and elective medication includes different modalities, each with its own proof base. Creating normalized conventions and rules that focus on wellbeing and viability is fundamental for the believability of all encompassing practices.

Interdisciplinary Coordinated effort:

All encompassing recuperating rehearses frequently include coordinated effort among different medical care experts, including traditional clinical professionals, corresponding advisors, and emotional wellness subject matter experts. Beating interdisciplinary obstructions and cultivating successful correspondence among assorted medical services groups present difficulties in the execution of comprehensive consideration models.

Procedures for Execution:

To effectively coordinate all encompassing mending rehearses in multispeciality emergency clinics, key execution is fundamental. These methodologies envelop a scope of drives that address social, underlying, and instructive parts of medical services conveyance.

Far reaching Preparing Projects:

Carrying out thorough preparation programs for medical services experts is critical. Preparing ought to cover the standards of all encompassing mending, relational abilities, and the protected mix of reciprocal treatments. Guaranteeing that medical services suppliers are knowledgeable in the proof base and advantages of comprehensive methodologies cultivates a more educated and cooperative consideration climate.

Production of All encompassing Recuperating Focuses:

Laying out committed comprehensive recuperating focuses inside multispeciality medical clinics gives an actual space to the combination of integral treatments. These focuses can offer various administrations, including needle therapy, back rub, reflection, and nourishing advising. Making a concentrated center point for comprehensive recuperating adds to the openness and perceivability of these practices.

Patient Schooling and Informed Assent:

Taking part in quiet schooling drives is fundamental for advancing comprehension and acknowledgment of all encompassing mending rehearses. Giving clear and straightforward data about the advantages, dangers, and proof base of reciprocal treatments enables patients to pursue informed choices. Informed assent processes guarantee that patients effectively partake in their consideration plans.

Examination and Result Estimation:

Putting resources into research drives to evaluate the viability of all encompassing mending rehearses adds to the proof base supporting their joining. Result estimation devices and exploration concentrates on assist with showing the effect of comprehensive methodologies on quiet results, fulfillment, and by and large prosperity. This exploration fabricates validity and illuminate constant improvement endeavors.

Institutional Strategies and Backing:

Creating institutional approaches that help the incorporation of comprehensive recuperating rehearses is key. These arrangements ought to frame the extent of all encompassing consideration, the capabilities of professionals, and wellbeing norms. Institutional help from medical clinic initiative builds up the obligation to all encompassing recuperating and works with a strong climate for execution.

Joint effort with Outer Accomplices:

Multispeciality medical clinics can work together with outer accomplices, including scholarly foundations, comprehensive wellbeing associations, and local area based experts. Laying out organizations permits medical clinics to take advantage of outside skill, keep up to date with progressions in comprehensive consideration, and extend the scope of administrations proposed to patients.

Nonstop Quality Improvement:

Executing a consistent quality improvement system guarantees continuous assessment and refinement of comprehensive mending rehearses. Normal evaluations of patient results, fulfillment studies, and criticism systems give significant bits of knowledge. Iterative upgrades in light of information add to the continuous advancement and streamlining of comprehensive consideration models.

5.1 Integrative Medicine Departments

The development of medical care has seen a change in outlook with the foundation of Integrative Medication Divisions inside clinical establishments. Integrative medication, a comprehensive methodology that joins customary clinical practices with proof based correlative treatments, is acquiring noticeable quality as a groundbreaking model of care. Integrative Medication Divisions assume a critical part in cultivating cooperation among medical services experts, tending to the different necessities of patients, and embracing a more understanding focused and exhaustive way to deal with prosperity. This investigation dives into the standards, advantages, difficulties, and procedures related with the foundation and working of Integrative Medication Divisions.

Standards of Integrative Medication Divisions:

Integrative Medication Divisions work in light of a bunch of central rules that guide their way to deal with patient consideration and health. These standards mirror a guarantee to joining the best of traditional medication with correlative treatments in a proof based and patient-focused way.

All encompassing Way to deal with Care:

At the center of integrative medication is a comprehensive methodology that perceives the interconnected idea of physical, mental, close to home, and profound prosperity. Integrative Medication Offices center around treating the entire individual as opposed to secluded side effects, taking into account way of life, sustenance, and psychosocial factors notwithstanding ailments.

Coordinated effort among Medical care Disciplines:

Integrative Medication Offices underline interdisciplinary coordinated effort, uniting medical services experts from different disciplines. This coordinated effort might incorporate clinical specialists, naturopathic doctors, acupuncturists, nutritionists, psychological wellness subject matter experts, and different professionals.

The objective is to use the mastery of different disciplines to give a thorough and coordinated way to deal with patient consideration.

Proof Based Practices:

Integrative Medication Divisions focus on proof based works on, guaranteeing that reciprocal treatments offered have a logical establishment and demonstrated viability. The incorporation of proof based correlative treatments close by ordinary medicines upgrades the general viability of patient consideration.

Patient-Focused Care:

Patient-focused care is a foundation of integrative medication. Integrative Medication Divisions effectively draw in patients in the dynamic cycle, taking into account their inclinations, values, and objectives. The cooperative association between medical care suppliers and patients engages people to effectively partake in their medical care venture.

Accentuation on Preventive Medication:

Integrative Medication Offices put a huge accentuation on preventive measures and way of life changes to advance long haul wellbeing. By tending to gamble with factors, advancing sound propensities, and offering preventive mediations, these divisions add to the anticipation of ongoing circumstances and the advancement of generally prosperity.

Advantages of Integrative Medication Divisions:

The foundation of Integrative Medication Divisions yields a large number of advantages that reach out to patients, medical services experts, and the medical care framework in general. These advantages add to worked on quiet results, upgraded fulfillment, and a more comprehensive way to deal with medical care conveyance.

Far reaching Patient Consideration:

Integrative Medication Divisions offer far reaching patient consideration that tends to the different requirements of people. By consolidating regular clinical medicines with integral treatments, these divisions give a range of restorative choices, guaranteeing that patients get customized and comprehensive consideration.

Upgraded Treatment Adequacy:

The reconciliation of proof based integral treatments close by traditional medicines can improve in general treatment adequacy. For specific circumstances, for example, constant agony, psychological wellness issues, and persistent sicknesses, the mix of treatments from different disciplines might bring about improved results contrasted with ordinary therapies alone.

Worked on Personal satisfaction:

Integrative Medication Divisions add to a superior personal satisfaction for patients by tending to their ailments as well as the more extensive parts of prosperity. Corresponding treatments, like needle therapy, back rub, and brain body rehearses, can decidedly influence close to home and psychological well-being, adding to an upgraded in general personal satisfaction.

Positive Patient Experience:

The patient-focused approach of Integrative Medication Divisions adds to a positive medical services insight. Patients value the customized care, the chance to effectively partake in direction, and the accessibility of correlative treatments that line up with their inclinations. Positive patient encounters are related with better adherence to treatment designs and further developed results.

Diminished Symptoms of Regular Medicines:

A few reciprocal treatments coordinated into patient consideration plans might assist with relieving the symptoms of customary clinical medicines. For example, needle therapy and brain body practices might help with overseeing treatment-related side effects like agony, queasiness, and weakness. This joining adds to a more adjusted and okay medical services insight.

Strengthening of Patients:

Integrative Medication Divisions engage patients to play a functioning job in their wellbeing and prosperity. Through training, shared navigation, and an emphasis on preventive measures, patients become accomplices in their medical care venture. This strengthening encourages a feeling of control and organization, decidedly impacting patient commitment and results.

Challenges in Laying out Integrative Medication Offices:

While the advantages are huge, the foundation and working of Integrative Medication Divisions face a few difficulties. Tending to these difficulties is fundamental for the effective reconciliation of reciprocal treatments inside the customary medical services system.

Social Shift inside Medical services Frameworks:

The reconciliation of integrative medication requires a social shift inside medical services frameworks. Protection from change, wariness among some medical care experts, and the requirement for thorough preparation present difficulties in encouraging a culture that embraces an integrative methodology.

Asset Designation and Financing:

Integrative Medication Offices might confront asset requirements and monetary difficulties. The designation of adequate assets to help preparing programs, the work of corresponding treatment professionals, and the production of devoted spaces for integrative consideration is fundamental. Getting assets and showing the expense adequacy of integrative methodologies are difficulties in numerous medical care settings.

Normalization and Credentialing:

Normalizing the act of integrative medication and laying out credentialing guidelines for reciprocal treatment professionals are difficulties. Guaranteeing that specialists meet laid out measures for capability and wellbeing is significant for the believability and viability of integrative consideration.

Interdisciplinary Cooperation:

Compelling joint effort among medical services experts from various disciplines is fundamental for the outcome of Integrative Medication Divisions. Defeating storehouses, encouraging correspondence, and making a common perspective of the objectives and advantages of integrative consideration are difficulties that require coordinated endeavors.

Systems for Execution:

To effectively lay out and work Integrative Medication Divisions, vital execution is fundamental. These systems envelop a scope of drives that address social, primary, and instructive parts of medical care conveyance.

Exhaustive Preparation Projects:

Executing exhaustive preparation programs for medical services experts is critical. Preparing ought to cover the standards of integrative medication, relational abilities, and the protected incorporation of correlative treatments. Guaranteeing that medical services suppliers are knowledgeable in the proof base and advantages of integrative methodologies cultivates a more educated and cooperative consideration climate.

Production of Integrative Medication Places:

Laying out committed Integrative Medication Places inside medical care foundations gives an actual space to the incorporation of reciprocal treatments. These focuses can offer various administrations, including needle therapy, knead, care programs, and nourishing advising. Making a unified center point for integrative medication adds to the openness and perceivability of these practices.

Patient Schooling and Informed Assent:

Participating in tolerant training drives is fundamental for advancing comprehension and acknowledgment of integrative medication rehearses. Giving clear and straightforward data about the advantages, dangers, and proof base of integral treatments engages patients to settle on informed choices. Informed assent processes guarantee that patients effectively partake in their consideration plans.

Exploration and Result Estimation:

Putting resources into research drives to survey the viability of integrative medication rehearses adds to the proof base supporting their coordination. Result estimation instruments and examination concentrates on assist with exhibiting the effect of integrative methodologies on tolerant results, fulfillment, and by and large prosperity. This examination fabricates validity and illuminate constant improvement endeavors.

Institutional Approaches and Backing:

Creating institutional approaches that help the reconciliation of integrative medication rehearses is major. These approaches ought to frame the extent of integrative consideration, the capabilities of specialists, and security norms. Institutional help from emergency clinic initiative builds up the obligation to integrative medication and works with a steady climate for execution.

Coordinated effort with Outer Accomplices:

Medical care foundations can work together with outer accomplices, including scholarly establishments, integrative medication associations, and local area based professionals. Laying out organizations permits establishments to take advantage of outer skill, keep up to date with headways in integrative consideration, and extend the scope of administrations proposed to patients.

Consistent Quality Improvement:

Carrying out a constant quality improvement structure guarantees progressing assessment and refinement of integrative medication rehearses. Standard evaluations of patient results, fulfillment reviews, and criticism components give significant bits of knowledge. Iterative upgrades in view of information add to the continuous advancement and enhancement of integrative consideration models.

5.2 Holistic Nursing Practices

All encompassing Nursing Works on: Sustaining Mending through Exhaustive Consideration

Comprehensive nursing rehearses address a groundbreaking way to deal with medical care that rises above the customary spotlight on actual side effects to embrace the interconnected elements of psyche, body, and soul. Established in the way of thinking that people are entire creatures with one of a kind requirements, all encompassing nursing underlines the significance of tending to the illness or disease as well as the more extensive parts of prosperity. This investigation dives into the standards, advantages, difficulties, and techniques related with all encompassing nursing works on, featuring their job in cultivating mending and upgrading the general patient experience.

Standards of All encompassing Nursing Practices:

All encompassing nursing rehearses are directed by a bunch of major rules that recognize them from customary medical care draws near. These standards highlight the significance of perceiving and tending to the multi-layered nature of people, recognizing the impact of mental, close to home, social, and profound variables on wellbeing.

Completeness and Uniqueness:

Comprehensive nursing sees people as entire creatures, considering their physical, mental, close to home, and profound aspects. This standard underscores the uniqueness of every individual, perceiving that medical services intercessions ought to be custom-made to the singular's particular necessities, inclinations, and values.

Comprehensive Appraisal:

All encompassing medical attendants take part in exhaustive appraisals that stretch out past actual side effects. They investigate patients' close to home states, social emotionally supportive networks, conviction frameworks, and way of life factors. This comprehensive evaluation empowers medical caretakers to acquire a more profound comprehension of the elements impacting a patient's wellbeing and prosperity.

Advancement of Self-Recuperating:

Comprehensive nursing rehearses focus on the natural limit with regards to self-mending inside people. Medical caretakers team up with patients to distinguish and improve their innate capacities to mend, encouraging a feeling of strengthening and dynamic support in the recuperating system.

All encompassing Correspondence:

Viable correspondence is integral to comprehensive nursing. All encompassing attendants take part in open and remedial correspondence that goes past passing on clinical data. They effectively tune in, approve patient encounters, and establish a sympathetic and strong climate that urges patients to share their interests and sentiments.

Mix of Corresponding Treatments:

All encompassing nursing embraces the incorporation of corresponding treatments close by traditional clinical medicines. These may incorporate modalities, for example, restorative touch, fragrance based treatment, care rehearses, and healthful direction. The objective is to offer a different scope of mediations that address the assorted requirements of patients.

Advantages of Comprehensive Nursing Practices:

The reception of comprehensive nursing rehearses yields a horde of advantages that reach out to patients, medical care experts, and the medical services framework. These advantages add to worked on understanding results, improved fulfillment, and a more merciful and customized way to deal with care.

Worked on Tolerant Prosperity:

All encompassing nursing rehearses add to the general prosperity of patients by tending to their actual infirmities as well as their close to home and profound requirements. This exhaustive methodology encourages a feeling of completeness and supports patients in accomplishing a more excellent of life.

Upgraded Patient-Supplier Relationship:

The patient-supplier relationship is fortified through comprehensive nursing rehearses. By recognizing the uniqueness of patients and participating in open correspondence, comprehensive medical caretakers fabricate trust and compatibility. A positive and cooperative relationship adds to worked on persistent fulfillment and adherence to treatment plans.

Diminished Pressure and Nervousness:

Comprehensive nursing intercessions, like unwinding strategies, directed symbolism, and care rehearses, add to the decrease of pressure and nervousness levels among patients. By tending to profound and mental viewpoints, all encompassing nursing rehearses establish a remedial climate that upholds mental prosperity.

Exhaustive Agony The executives:

All encompassing medical caretakers utilize a scope of integral treatments to address torment and uneasiness. Methods like restorative touch, needle therapy, and back rub might be incorporated into torment the executives plans, offering patients extra devices for adapting to torment past traditional prescriptions.

Strengthening of Patients:

All encompassing nursing rehearses engage patients to effectively take part in their medical care venture. By including patients in direction, giving schooling about taking care of oneself practices, and empowering way of life changes, all encompassing medical caretakers cultivate a feeling of strengthening that emphatically impacts patient commitment and results.

Challenges in Executing All encompassing Nursing Practices:

While the advantages are significant, the coordination of all encompassing nursing rehearses faces difficulties inside the medical care scene. Beating these difficulties requires a coordinated work to move standards, give schooling, and encourage a culture that embraces all encompassing methodologies.

Social Shift inside Medical care Frameworks:

The reception of all encompassing nursing rehearses requires a social shift inside medical services frameworks. Protection from change, doubt among some medical services experts, and the requirement for complete preparation present difficulties in encouraging a culture that qualities and coordinates comprehensive consideration.

Time Limitations and Responsibility:

All encompassing nursing practices might call for extra investment for exhaustive evaluations, restorative correspondence, and the coordination of reciprocal treatments. Time imperatives and weighty jobs in medical services settings might present difficulties to the compelling execution of all encompassing consideration rehearses.

Coordination into Conventional Consideration Models:

Coordinating all encompassing nursing rehearses into customary consideration models can challenge. Medical services organizations might have to rethink existing consideration designs, strategies, and work processes to oblige the all encompassing methodology. Adjusting all encompassing practices to customary consideration while keeping up with productivity is a fragile equilibrium.

Normalization and Training:

Normalizing all encompassing nursing rehearses and giving schooling to medical services experts are fundamental difficulties. Laying out clear rules, conventions, and instructive projects guarantees that comprehensive consideration is conveyed reliably and securely across different medical care settings.

Procedures for Execution:

To effectively carry out comprehensive nursing rehearses, key drives are required. These techniques incorporate a scope of measures that address social, instructive, and underlying parts of medical services conveyance.

Exhaustive Preparation Projects:

Executing far reaching preparing programs for medical attendants and medical services experts is significant. Preparing ought to cover the standards of comprehensive nursing, successful relational abilities, and the protected reconciliation of corresponding treatments. Guaranteeing that medical services suppliers are exceptional with the information and abilities required for comprehensive consideration is fundamental.

Making of All encompassing Nursing Units or Groups:

Laying out devoted all encompassing nursing units or groups inside medical services foundations gives an engaged climate to the conveyance of comprehensive consideration. These units can act as trailblazers in the mix of comprehensive works on, encouraging a culture that upholds the standards of all encompassing nursing.

Patient Training and Informed Assent:

Participating in quiet schooling drives is fundamental for advancing comprehension and acknowledgment of all encompassing nursing rehearses. Giving clear data about the advantages, dangers, and proof base of all encompassing mediations enables patients to effectively partake in their consideration plans. Informed assent processes guarantee that patients are very much educated and taken part in their comprehensive consideration.

Exploration and Result Estimation:

Putting resources into research drives to survey the viability of comprehensive nursing rehearses adds to the proof base supporting their mix. Result estimation devices and examination concentrates on assist with exhibiting the effect of all encompassing methodologies on tolerant results, fulfillment, and generally prosperity. This examination effectively assembles believability and illuminate persistent improvement endeavors.

Institutional Approaches and Backing:

Creating institutional strategies that help the reconciliation of comprehensive nursing rehearses is essential. These approaches ought to frame the extent of comprehensive consideration, the capabilities of all encompassing nursing specialists, and security principles. Institutional help from nursing initiative and medical care overseers builds up the obligation to comprehensive nursing and establishes a steady climate for execution.

5.3 Holistic Rehabilitation Programs

All encompassing Restoration Projects: Changing Lives through Exhaustive Recuperation

Comprehensive restoration programs address a creative and extraordinary way to deal with the recuperation interaction, tending to not just the actual parts of a singular's condition yet in addition the profound, mental, and otherworldly aspects. Established in the way of thinking that people are mind boggling creatures with interconnected needs, comprehensive restoration perceives the significance of getting the entire individual accomplish enduring recuperation. This investigation dives into the standards, advantages, difficulties, and techniques related with all encompassing restoration programs, featuring their part in cultivating far reaching recuperating and upgrading the general prosperity of people on their recuperation process.

Standards of Comprehensive Recovery Projects:

Comprehensive restoration programs are directed by a bunch of fundamental rules that underline the significance of tending to all features of a singular's life during the recuperation interaction.

Thorough Evaluation:

All encompassing restoration starts with a complete evaluation that goes past the distinguishing proof of actual side effects. Appraisals think about the person's emotional wellness, close to home prosperity, social emotionally supportive networks, and profound convictions. This comprehensive methodology makes a custom-made and individualized recuperation plan.

Tending to the Main drivers:

Comprehensive restoration perceives that habit and psychological well-being difficulties frequently have basic underlying drivers. These projects expect to recognize and address the underlying drivers of people's battles, whether they are connected with injury, irritating intense subject matters, or different elements adding to their condition.

Integrative Treatments:

All encompassing restoration programs coordinate different helpful modalities past conventional methodologies. These may incorporate care rehearses, yoga, workmanship treatment, music treatment, and other corresponding treatments that advance mending on different levels.

Mind-Body Association:

Comprehensive restoration stresses the interconnectedness of the psyche and body. Perceiving the effect of mental and profound prosperity on actual wellbeing, these projects integrate mediations that help the psyche body association, like reflection, breathwork, and stress-decrease strategies.

Customized Treatment Plans:

Comprehensive restoration perceives that every individual's excursion to recuperation is one of a kind. Treatment plans are customized to address the particular requirements, inclinations, and objectives of the person. This individualized methodology cultivates a feeling of strengthening and dynamic cooperation in the recuperation cycle.

Advantages of All encompassing Recovery Projects:

The reception of all encompassing restoration programs achieves a scope of advantages that add to further developed results and the general prosperity of people looking for recuperation.

Thorough Recuperating:

All encompassing restoration programs focus on exhaustive recuperating by tending to the physical, mental, close to home, and otherworldly parts of a singular's life. This approach goes past side effect the board to focus on the basic reasons for enslavement or emotional well-being difficulties, advancing enduring recuperation.

Improved Mindfulness:

All encompassing recovery urges people to foster an increased identity mindfulness. Through remedial modalities like care and self-reflection, people gain experiences into their thinking examples, feelings, and ways of behaving. This expanded mindfulness is an incredible asset for supported recuperation.

Worked on Mental and Close to home Prosperity:

Comprehensive recovery programs add to worked on mental and profound prosperity by tending to psychological well-being concerns, injury, and inner difficulties. Restorative mediations center around building adapting abilities, strength, and profound guideline, cultivating a positive effect on generally emotional wellness.

Strengthening and Self-Viability:

Comprehensive restoration puts areas of strength for an on strengthening and self-viability. By including people in the co-production of their treatment designs and giving devices to taking care of oneself, these projects engage people to play a functioning job in their recuperation process, upgrading their feeling of control and certainty.

Comprehensive Emotionally supportive network:

Comprehensive restoration programs perceive the significance of social help in the recuperation cycle. These projects frequently integrate bunch treatment, family treatment, and companion backing to make an all encompassing emotionally supportive network. Building associations with other people who share comparable encounters cultivates a feeling of local area and understanding.

Challenges in Executing Comprehensive Restoration Projects:

The execution of comprehensive recovery programs isn't without challenges. Conquering these moves requires a pledge to moving ideal models, tending to social boundaries, and incorporating comprehensive methodologies into the current medical care structure.

Incorporation into Customary Models:

All encompassing recovery projects might confront opposition while incorporating into conventional models of enslavement treatment or psychological well-being care. Moving from an exclusively clinical or social model to an all encompassing methodology requires a social shift inside medical services frameworks.

Staff Preparing and Schooling:

Medical services experts working in recovery settings might require extra preparation and training to successfully comprehend and execute all encompassing methodologies. This remembers preparing for corresponding treatments, all encompassing evaluation procedures, and the standards of psyche body medication.

Asset Designation:

Comprehensive recovery projects might confront asset imperatives, remembering monetary contemplations and limits for staffing. Distributing assets for the reconciliation of corresponding treatments, comprehensive appraisals, and individualized treatment plans is fundamental for the progress of these projects.

Estimating Comprehensive Results:

Customary result measures may not completely catch the comprehensive advantages of recovery programs. Creating and carrying out measures that survey mental, profound, and otherworldly prosperity close by customary measurements is a test that requires cautious thought.

Systems for Execution:

To effectively execute all encompassing recovery programs, vital drives are essential. These systems include a scope of measures that address social, instructive, and underlying parts of medical care conveyance.

Thorough Staff Preparing:

Carrying out complete preparation programs for medical services experts is critical. This preparing ought to cover the standards of comprehensive restoration, successful relational abilities, and the protected reconciliation of reciprocal treatments. Guaranteeing that medical services suppliers are exceptional with the information and abilities required for all encompassing consideration is fundamental.

Comprehensive Program Coordination:

Laying out committed comprehensive recovery projects or units inside medical services foundations gives an engaged climate to the conveyance of all encompassing consideration. These projects can act as trailblazers in the coordination of all encompassing works on, cultivating a culture that upholds the standards of comprehensive recovery.

Individualized Treatment Plans:

All encompassing recovery underlines the significance of customized and individualized treatment plans. Medical care experts ought to team up with people in the co-formation of their recuperation plans, considering their remarkable necessities, inclinations, and objectives.

Integrating Innovation:

Utilizing innovation can improve the availability and conveyance of all encompassing recovery administrations. Virtual stages, versatile applications, and telehealth administrations can be incorporated to offer continuous help, instruction, and remedial intercessions.

Local area Associations:

All encompassing restoration projects can profit from shaping associations with local area associations, comprehensive wellbeing specialists, and care groups. These organizations extend the scope of administrations offered and make a more far reaching and interconnected organization of help for people in recuperation.

Chapter 6

Successful Implementation

The effective execution of all encompassing recovery programs requires a key and smart methodology that addresses social, instructive, and primary perspectives inside medical care frameworks. By perceiving the interconnected idea of physical, mental, profound, and otherworldly prosperity, these projects expect to cultivate enduring recuperation and work on the general personal satisfaction for people. This investigation dives into key systems for the effective execution of comprehensive recovery programs, recognizing the difficulties and illustrating the rules that guide their combination into the current medical services structure.

Standards Directing Effective Execution:

Social Shift towards Comprehensive Consideration:

The establishment for effective execution lies in cultivating a social shift inside medical care frameworks. This includes developing a climate that qualities and focuses on all encompassing consideration, perceiving its job in working on understanding results and by and large prosperity. Administration support, instructive drives, and open correspondence add to making a culture that embraces all encompassing recovery.

Interdisciplinary Joint effort:

All encompassing recovery programs blossom with interdisciplinary cooperation. Fruitful execution includes separating storehouses and cultivating correspondence among medical services experts from assorted disciplines. This joint effort guarantees that the interesting necessities of people are tended to completely, drawing on the skill of clinical, mental, and corresponding treatment professionals.

Individualized Treatment Arranging:

A foundation of effective execution is the turn of events and execution of individualized treatment plans. Perceiving that every individual's excursion to recuperation is extraordinary, these plans ought to be custom-made to address the particular physical, mental, and close to home necessities of people. The cooperative making of these plans engages people to effectively partake in their recuperation cycle.

Complete Staff Preparing:

Effective execution requires medical services experts to go through thorough preparation in the standards of comprehensive consideration. Preparing projects ought to cover all encompassing evaluation procedures, compelling relational abilities, and the protected mix of reciprocal treatments. Thoroughly prepared experts are fundamental for giving top caliber, individual focused care inside all encompassing restoration programs.

Patient Schooling and Commitment:

Drawing in patients in their consideration is crucial for effective execution. All encompassing restoration programs stress patient training, guaranteeing that people grasp the standards and advantages of comprehensive consideration. By effectively including patients in navigation and objective setting, these projects engage people to take responsibility for recuperation venture.

Procedures for Fruitful Execution:

Thorough Preparation Projects:

Carrying out thorough preparation programs for medical services experts is fundamental for effective joining. These projects ought to cover the standards of all encompassing consideration, compelling correspondence, and the protected execution of reciprocal treatments. Consistent expert improvement open doors guarantee that staff stays knowledgeable in all encompassing methodologies.

Making of Devoted Units:

Laying out devoted units or offices inside medical services foundations for all encompassing recovery establishes an engaged climate for effective execution. These units act as focuses of greatness, spearheading the combination of all encompassing practices and cultivating a culture that upholds the standards of comprehensive consideration.

Joint effort with All encompassing Wellbeing Experts:

Effective execution includes working together with comprehensive wellbeing specialists, including acupuncturists, rub advisors, yoga educators, and other corresponding treatment suppliers. Shaping organizations with these professionals grows the scope of administrations presented inside restoration programs and adds to a more comprehensive way to deal with care.

Joining of Innovation:

Utilizing innovation is an essential move for effective execution. Virtual stages, telehealth administrations, and versatile applications can upgrade the availability of all encompassing restoration administrations. These advances work with progressing backing, training, and remedial intercessions, beating hindrances of distance and upgrading in general program viability.

Local area Commitment and Organizations:

Comprehensive recovery programs benefit from drawing in with the local area and framing associations with neighborhood associations. These organizations give extra assets, encouraging groups of people, and roads for local area based exercises that supplement the all encompassing methodology. Connecting with the local area encourages a feeling of having a place and backing for people in recuperation.

Checking and Consistent Improvement:

Carrying out a strong observing and consistent improvement structure is fundamental for progress. Ordinary appraisals of patient results, program viability, and staff fulfillment add to continuous refinement and improvement. A pledge to information driven navigation guarantees that the program develops to meet the changing necessities of the people it serves.

Schooling and Mindfulness Missions:

Making mindfulness about comprehensive restoration programs is urgent for fruitful execution. Schooling efforts focusing on both medical care experts and the local area assist with dissipating confusions, assemble understanding, and produce support. By advancing the standards and advantages of all encompassing consideration, these missions add to a positive gathering and commitment with the projects.

Difficulties and Alleviation Systems:

Protection from Social Shift:

Protection from a social shift towards comprehensive consideration might emerge from dug in practices and convictions. Alleviation includes clear correspondence about the advantages of all encompassing restoration, displaying examples of overcoming adversity, and including key partners in the dynamic cycle. Authority backing and job displaying assume a critical part in beating obstruction.

Asset Imperatives:

Asset imperatives, including monetary contemplations and staffing restrictions, present difficulties for effective execution. Relief methodologies include pushing for asset portion, showing the expense viability of comprehensive methodologies, and investigating imaginative subsidizing arrangements. Exhibiting the positive effect on tolerant results can accumulate support for asset portion.

Normalization and Credentialing:

Normalizing the act of comprehensive recovery and laying out credentialing principles for integral treatment professionals are difficulties. Alleviation includes making progress toward agreement inside the medical services local area, growing clear rules, and teaming up with certifying bodies. Laying out thorough guidelines guarantees the wellbeing and adequacy of comprehensive consideration rehearses.

Estimating Comprehensive Results:

Conventional result measures may not completely catch the comprehensive advantages of restoration programs. Alleviation includes the turn of events and execution of result estimates that evaluate mental, profound, and otherworldly prosperity close by customary measurements. Cooperation with scientists and specialists in result estimation upgrades the legitimacy of these actions.

6.1 Examples of Multispeciality Hospitals Embracing Holistic Healing

Instances of Multispeciality Emergency clinics Embracing All encompassing Mending: Spearheading Complete Patient Consideration

Lately, a rising number of multispeciality medical clinics have perceived the worth of all encompassing recuperating approaches in giving extensive and patient-focused care. These medical clinics are splitting away from customary models and coordinating correlative treatments, mind-body rehearses, and all encompassing ways of thinking into their medical services administrations. This investigation features instances of multispeciality clinics that have effectively embraced comprehensive mending, setting new norms for patient consideration and prosperity.

Cleveland Facility's Middle for Integrative Medication:

The Cleveland Facility, eminent for its obligation to clinical advancement, houses the Middle for Integrative Medication. This middle is a brilliant illustration of how a multispeciality medical clinic can integrate all encompassing mending into its contributions. The Middle for Integrative Medication gives a scope of administrations, including needle therapy, knead treatment, care based pressure decrease, and wholesome directing. By coordinating these integral treatments with traditional clinical medicines, the Cleveland Facility intends to address the physical, mental, and profound components of patient wellbeing, offering a more exhaustive and patient-focused approach.

Mayo Center's Correlative and Integrative Medication Program:

The Mayo Center, known for its greatness in medical care, has embraced all encompassing mending through its Corresponding and Integrative Medication Program. This program coordinates proof based integral treatments into the general consideration plans for patients. Instances of administrations offered incorporate needle therapy, chiropractic care, knead treatment, and integrative oncology. By consolidating these treatments, the Mayo Facility plans to upgrade the general prosperity of patients and further develop treatment results, perceiving the significance of tending to the brain body association in medical services.

Johns Hopkins Integrative Medication and Stomach related Center:

Johns Hopkins Medication has laid out the Integrative Medication and Stomach related Center, exhibiting a pledge to all encompassing mending. This middle spotlights on giving integrative consideration to patients with stomach related messes, perceiving the effect of way of life, stress, and close to home prosperity on gastrointestinal wellbeing. The middle offers administrations, for example, needle therapy, mind-body treatments, and healthful guiding. By recognizing the interconnected idea of physical and profound wellbeing, Johns Hopkins Medication shows how multispeciality clinics can fit all encompassing ways to deal with address explicit ailments.

MD Anderson Disease Center's Integrative Medication Program:

The MD Anderson Malignant growth Community, a main organization in disease care, has consolidated comprehensive mending through its Integrative Medication Program. Perceiving the special difficulties looked by malignant growth patients, this program offers a scope of integral treatments, including needle therapy, back rub, yoga, and reflection. These treatments are coordinated into malignant growth therapy intends to assist with overseeing side effects, work on personal satisfaction, and address the all encompassing requirements of patients going through disease care. MD Anderson's methodology exhibits how multispeciality clinics can improve the disease patient's process by integrating comprehensive standards into oncology care.

Brigham and Ladies' Emergency clinic's Osher Clinical Community for Integrative Medication:

The Osher Clinical Place for Integrative Medication at Brigham and Ladies' Medical clinic is a striking illustration of a multispeciality medical clinic embracing all encompassing mending. This middle offers different integrative treatments, including needle therapy, mind-body treatments, and dietary directing. The emphasis is on giving customized care that thinks about the entire individual and underscores patient strengthening. By incorporating these all encompassing methodologies, Brigham and Ladies' Clinic embodies how multispeciality organizations can make focuses of greatness devoted to far reaching patient consideration.

Stanford Medical services' Middle for Integrative Medication:

Stanford Medical services has laid out the Middle for Integrative Medication, showing a guarantee to joining customary medication with all encompassing methodologies. The middle offers administrations like needle therapy, integrative oncology, and brain body rehearses. Stanford's methodology underlines the joining of proof based reciprocal treatments to upgrade patient results, oversee side effects, and work on generally prosperity. The consideration of integrative oncology features the acknowledgment of all encompassing recuperating with regards to malignant growth care.

Duke Integrative Medication at Duke College Wellbeing Framework:

Duke Integrative Medication, part of the Duke College Wellbeing Framework, is a thorough illustration of a multispeciality emergency clinic embracing comprehensive recuperating. The middle offers a scope of administrations, including integrative wellbeing instructing, needle therapy, and brain body programs. Duke Integrative Medication centers around enabling people to play a functioning job in their wellbeing and prosperity. By incorporating these administrations, Duke College Wellbeing Framework exhibits a promise to a patient-focused and comprehensive way to deal with medical services.

Repeating themes Among Models:

These models share consistent ideas that feature the vital standards and systems utilized by multispeciality medical clinics embracing comprehensive mending:

Interdisciplinary Joint effort:

Every one of these emergency clinics stresses interdisciplinary joint effort, uniting medical services experts from assorted claims to fame. This cooperative methodology guarantees that patients get far reaching care that addresses their physical, mental, and close to home prosperity.

Customized and Patient-Focused Care:

All encompassing recuperating in these emergency clinics is established in customized and patient-focused care. Treatment plans are customized to individual necessities, inclinations, and objectives, perceiving that every individual's excursion to wellbeing is interesting.

Joining of Corresponding Treatments:

Reciprocal treatments, like needle therapy, back rub, yoga, and brain body rehearses, are coordinated close by customary clinical medicines. This reconciliation upgrades the general consideration gave, tending to a more extensive range of patient requirements.

Center around Health and Anticipation:

All encompassing mending reaches out past the treatment of sickness to zero in on wellbeing and anticipation. These clinics perceive the significance of way of life factors, stress the board, and profound prosperity in keeping up with by and large wellbeing and forestalling sickness.

Exploration and Proof Based Practices:

A large number of these models consolidate proof based works on, underscoring the significance of exploration in supporting the combination of comprehensive methodologies. Research drives add to the developing assemblage of proof supporting the adequacy of correlative treatments in medical services.

6.2 Impact on Patient Outcomes and Satisfaction

Influence on Tolerant Results and Fulfillment: All encompassing Mending in Multispeciality Medical clinics

The reconciliation of all encompassing mending approaches inside multispeciality medical clinics has significant ramifications for patient results and fulfillment. Past the customary spotlight on treating illnesses and side effects, comprehensive recuperating perceives the interconnected elements of physical, mental, close to home, and profound prosperity. This investigation dives into the effect of all encompassing recuperating on persistent results and fulfillment, featuring how a thorough way to deal with medical care changes the patient experience.

Upgraded Patient Results:

Thorough Mending:

All encompassing mending targets tending to the underlying drivers of medical problems, as opposed to just easing side effects. By taking into account the entire individual — brain, body, and soul — multispeciality clinics utilizing all encompassing methodologies add to thorough recuperating. This comprehensive point of view frequently prompts worked on persistent results, as hidden issues are distinguished and tended to, advancing supported prosperity.

Further developed Ongoing Sickness The board:

For patients with constant illnesses, comprehensive mending offers a multi-layered approach. Reciprocal treatments like needle therapy, yoga, and care practices might be incorporated into therapy plans, improving the viability of customary clinical mediations. This coordinated methodology frequently brings about better administration of ongoing circumstances, further developed side effect control, and upgraded generally personal satisfaction for patients.

Diminished Treatment-Related Incidental effects:

Comprehensive methodologies, for example, integrative oncology in disease care, have shown an ability to decrease treatment-related secondary effects. Methods like needle therapy and psyche body rehearses add to overseeing side effects like agony, queasiness, and exhaustion. Thus, patients going through customary clinical medicines experience a more excellent of life and are better ready to endure the afflictions of their helpful regimens.

Supporting Psychological well-being and Personal Prosperity:

All encompassing mending recognizes the perplexing association between emotional well-being and actual prosperity. Consolidating psychological wellness backing, advising, and mind-body rehearses inside multispeciality clinics emphatically influences patient results. Patients encountering emotional well-being difficulties frequently track down alleviation through all encompassing methodologies, prompting worked on profound prosperity and, thusly, upgraded generally wellbeing results.

Strengthening and Dynamic Patient Interest:

All encompassing recuperating puts areas of strength for an on engaging patients to effectively take part in their medical services venture. Patients are urged to participate in navigation, put forth private objectives, and take responsibility for prosperity. This dynamic cooperation adds to a feeling of strengthening, cultivating a good mentality that can fundamentally influence treatment adherence and generally wellbeing results.

Raised Patient Fulfillment:

Patient-Focused Care:

Comprehensive mending lines up with the standards of patient-focused care, putting the person at the focal point of medical services choices. Multispeciality emergency clinics embracing comprehensive methodologies focus on the extraordinary necessities, inclinations, and upsides of every patient. This patient-driven center upgrades fulfillment by making a medical services experience customized to the individual, cultivating a feeling of being seen and heard.

Further developed Correspondence and Trust:

The combination of all encompassing recuperating frequently includes further developed correspondence between medical services suppliers and patients. All encompassing methodologies underline open exchange, undivided attention, and a cooperative way to deal with direction. This improved correspondence fabricates trust among patients and medical services suppliers, adding to more significant levels of fulfillment with the consideration got.

Positive Medical care Climate:

All encompassing recuperating in multispeciality clinics frequently stretches out past clinical medicines to establish a positive and mending climate. Incorporating components like normal light, calming style, and spaces for unwinding adds to a more lovely and steady environment. Patients encountering an all encompassing medical care climate frequently report more elevated levels of fulfillment with their general clinic experience.

Consistent encouragement and Sympathy:

Comprehensive recuperating perceives the significance of basic reassurance and merciful consideration. Medical care suppliers consolidating all encompassing methodologies frequently invest extra energy with patients, tending to close to home worries and giving a listening ear. This sympathetic methodology adds to a more sure quiet insight and more significant levels of fulfillment with the consistent reassurance got during the medical services venture.

Customized and Comprehensive Training:

All encompassing recuperating includes instructing patients about the interconnected idea of their wellbeing. This instruction enables patients with information about way of life factors, taking care of oneself practices, and correlative treatments that can uphold their prosperity. Patients who get customized and comprehensive training frequently express more elevated levels of fulfillment, feeling more educated and effectively participated in their wellbeing.

Difficulties and Contemplations:

Social Shift and Obstruction:

The combination of all encompassing mending inside multispeciality emergency clinics might experience obstruction because of dug in social standards and customary medical care ideal models. Defeating this challenge requires a purposeful work to instruct medical services experts, heads, and the more extensive local area about the advantages and proof supporting comprehensive methodologies.

Asset Allotment:

Carrying out comprehensive mending practices might present difficulties connected with asset allotment, including financing and staffing contemplations. Exhibiting the expense viability and positive effect on tolerant results is fundamental for getting the important assets and backing for comprehensive drives.

Normalization and Preparing:

Normalizing all encompassing mending rehearses and guaranteeing that medical care experts are enough prepared in these methodologies are basic contemplations. Laying out clear rules, conventions, and preparing programs adds to the protected and powerful execution of comprehensive mending inside multispeciality emergency clinics.

Mix with Traditional Medication:

Blending all encompassing recuperating with traditional clinical practices requires cautious reconciliation. Multispeciality clinics need to find some kind of harmony between offering reciprocal treatments and guaranteeing the wellbeing and viability of these mediations inside the setting of regular clinical medicines.

6.3 Lessons Learned from Real-world Experiences

Examples Gained from True Encounters: Exploring the Combination of All encompassing Mending in Multispeciality Clinics

As multispeciality clinics proceed to investigate and incorporate comprehensive recuperating into their practices, significant illustrations rise up out of true encounters.

These illustrations, drawn from the difficulties and triumphs experienced in assorted medical services settings, give bits of knowledge into the intricacies of consolidating comprehensive methodologies inside ordinary clinical structures. This investigation dives into key illustrations mastered, offering direction for medical care experts, chairmen, and policymakers exploring the reconciliation of all encompassing mending in multispeciality clinics.

Patient-Focused Correspondence is Principal:

One of the focal examples learned is the basic significance of patient-focused correspondence. Successful correspondence that includes undivided attention, compassion, and a cooperative methodology fundamentally influences patient fulfillment and results. Comprehensive recuperating stresses the patient's exceptional necessities and inclinations, and medical services experts should focus on clear and open correspondence to fabricate trust and work with shared navigation.

Coordinated effort Across Disciplines is Fundamental:

Fruitful reconciliation of comprehensive mending requires joint effort across different medical care disciplines. Illustrations from genuine encounters underscore the requirement for a multidisciplinary approach where experts from different claims to fame cooperate flawlessly. This joint effort guarantees exhaustive consideration as well as encourages a climate where the advantages of both regular and all encompassing practices can be utilized for ideal patient results.

Customization is Key in All encompassing Consideration Plans:

Certifiable encounters feature the significance of customization in all encompassing consideration plans. Perceiving that every patient's process is exceptional, fitting intercessions to individual necessities, inclinations, and social foundations upgrades the viability of comprehensive mending. A one-size-fits-all approach doesn't line up with the standards of all encompassing consideration, and illustrations learned underline the worth of customized, patient-focused treatment plans.

Staff Preparing is a Nonstop Cycle:

The effective incorporation of all encompassing recuperating requires progressing staff preparing and schooling. Genuine encounters highlight that preparing medical care experts in comprehensive methodologies is certainly not a one-time exertion yet a nonstop cycle. This incorporates keeping up to date with arising research, refining abilities in corresponding treatments, and developing a mentality that embraces the standards of comprehensive mending.

Embracing Innovation Upgrades Access:

Illustrations learned uncover the job of innovation in improving admittance to comprehensive mending rehearses. Virtual stages, telehealth administrations, and versatile applications assume a vital part in expanding the range of all encompassing medical services past clinic walls. Coordinating innovation works with continuous patient help, schooling, and the conveyance of comprehensive mediations, especially in circumstances where in-person visits might challenge.

Tending to Staff Burnout and Prosperity is Significant:

The incorporation of all encompassing mending additionally focuses on the prosperity of medical care experts. Examples gained from true encounters underline the significance of tending to staff burnout and advancing their prosperity. Comprehensive methodologies shouldn't simply be applied to patient consideration yet additionally stretched out to help the psychological, close to home, and actual wellbeing of medical care suppliers.

Social Skill is a Foundation:

Perceiving and regarding social variety is a foundation of effective comprehensive mending incorporation. True encounters highlight the requirement for social capability among medical care experts. Grasping assorted conviction frameworks, customs, and practices is fundamental for giving comprehensive and powerful all encompassing consideration that regards the qualities and foundations of every patient.

Exploration and Proof Based Practice Fortify Validity:

Examples learned feature the meaning of examination and proof based practice in fortifying the validity of comprehensive mending. Thorough exploration drives add to the developing collection of proof supporting the adequacy of integral treatments and all encompassing methodologies. Genuine encounters underscore the significance of directing examinations to evaluate the effect of all encompassing mediations on understanding results, fulfillment, and generally speaking prosperity.

Adjusting Custom and Development is a Fragile Demonstration:

Coordinating comprehensive mending inside multispeciality clinics requires a fragile harmony among custom and development. Certifiable encounters exhibit that respecting laid out clinical practices while integrating creative all encompassing methodologies is fundamental. Finding some kind of harmony guarantees that patients get the advantages of both reliable and arising restorative modalities.

Patient Instruction is Engaging:

Teaching patients about all encompassing recuperating standards, rehearses, and the reasoning behind integrative consideration is enabling. Illustrations from genuine encounters pressure the significance of straightforward and patient-accommodating training. At the point when patients comprehend the all encompassing parts of their consideration, they are bound to effectively participate in the recuperating system and settle on informed conclusions about their wellbeing.

Adaptability and Flexibility are Vital:

The unique idea of medical care conditions requires adaptability and versatility in the joining of all encompassing recuperating. Certifiable encounters underline that medical services organizations should be receptive to advancing patient requirements, arising exploration, and changes in medical care scenes. A culture of flexibility guarantees that comprehensive methodologies stay significant and powerful in the steadily developing medical care scene.

Tending to All encompassing Recuperating Shame is a Persistent Exertion:

Defeating disgrace related with comprehensive mending requires a persistent exertion. Genuine illustrations instruct us that while acknowledgment of comprehensive methodologies is developing, challenges connected with wariness and misinterpretations endure. Endeavors to teach both medical care experts and people in general about the proof based nature of numerous all encompassing practices add to separating obstructions and cultivating acknowledgment.

Chapter 7

Challenges and Solutions

The mix of all encompassing mending into the texture of multispeciality medical clinics is a groundbreaking excursion that presents an interesting arrangement of difficulties. As medical services foundations endeavor to give more complete and patient-focused care, they experience hindrances connected with social movements, asset allotment, staff preparing, and the conjunction of conventional and all encompassing practices. This investigation dives into the difficulties looked in the coordination of all encompassing mending and proposes answers for explore these intricacies successfully.

Challenges:

Social Shift and Opposition:

Coordinating all encompassing recuperating requires an essential social shift inside medical care foundations. The conventional clinical model, established in proof based rehearses and laid out conventions, may experience opposition when stood up to with the all encompassing worldview. Distrust among medical care experts, managers, and even patients can impede the consistent consolidation of all encompassing methodologies into multispeciality clinics.

Asset Portion Imperatives:

Asset portion, including monetary contemplations and staffing restrictions, represents a critical test. Incorporating comprehensive recuperating frequently requires extra assets for preparing, framework, and corresponding treatment administrations. In a climate where spending plans are as of now extended meager, getting assets for all encompassing drives might be met with delay and contending needs.

Staff Preparing and Training:

Medical care experts might need openness to comprehensive mending during their proper training, prompting a hole in information and abilities. Coordinating integral treatments, mind-body rehearses, and comprehensive standards requires broad staff preparing. Be that as it may, the time imperatives and requests of day to day medical care activities make it trying to give thorough and progressing preparing to all staff individuals.

Normalization and Credentialing:

The normalization of comprehensive mending rehearses and the credentialing of integral treatment experts present difficulties. Dissimilar to traditional clinical medicines with laid out conventions, all encompassing methodologies might need all around perceived norms. This absence of normalization can prompt fluctuation in the nature of care gave and raises worries about quiet wellbeing.

Coordination with Ordinary Medication:

The amicable coordination of comprehensive methodologies with ordinary medication is a sensitive demonstration. Finding some kind of harmony to guarantee patient security, staying away from clashes among medicines, and keeping a durable patient consideration experience is testing. The concurrence of two standards, each with its own standards and methods of reasoning, requires smart route to make a consistent and correlative way to deal with medical services.

Arrangements:

Social Shift and Training Drives:

Addressing social protection from all encompassing recuperating includes strong training drives. Leading mindfulness crusades, giving proof based data, and displaying examples of overcoming adversity can assist with moving discernments. Empowering open exchanges about the advantages of all encompassing methodologies cultivates a culture of understanding and acknowledgment inside the medical services local area.

Support for Asset Allotment:

To beat asset portion requirements, medical care organizations need to present a convincing defense for the advantages of all encompassing mending. Showing the expense viability, positive effect on quiet results, and arrangement with patient-focused care standards can accumulate support from partners and legitimize the designation of assets for all encompassing drives.

Extensive Staff Preparing Projects:

Laying out extensive and continuous staff preparing programs is fundamental for effective incorporation. These projects ought to cover the standards of comprehensive mending, proof based integral treatments, and compelling relational abilities. Preparing ought to be customized to various jobs inside the medical services group, guaranteeing that all staff individuals are prepared to add to an all encompassing consideration climate.

Advancement of Clear Rules and Conventions:

Normalizing all encompassing recuperating rehearses requires the advancement of clear rules and conventions. Medical care foundations can team up with specialists in all encompassing ways to deal with lay out proof based principles for reciprocal treatments. Clear rules add to consistency by and by, improve patient security, and address concerns connected with the absence of normalization.

Interdisciplinary Coordinated effort:

Advancing interdisciplinary cooperation is critical to incorporating all encompassing methodologies with customary medication. Laying out ordinary discussions for medical services experts from different disciplines to team up, share experiences, and foster strong therapy plans improves correspondence and encourages a culture of collaboration. Cooperative consideration models that include both regular and all encompassing specialists add to a more exhaustive patient consideration experience.

Patient-Focused Relational abilities Preparing:

Improving patient-focused relational abilities is urgent for medical services experts engaged with comprehensive consideration. Preparing projects ought to zero in on undivided attention, compassion, and viable correspondence of comprehensive standards. Further developed correspondence guarantees that patients are very much educated, effectively participated in their consideration, and feel upheld in their all encompassing recuperating venture.

Advancement of Integrative Medication Divisions:

Making devoted integrative medication offices inside multispeciality clinics gives an engaged climate to all encompassing consideration. These divisions act as center points for ability in correlative treatments, comprehensive appraisals, and cooperative consideration arranging. Integrative medication divisions can spearhead the incorporation of comprehensive mending, exhibiting its viability and advancing a culture of all encompassing consideration inside the bigger organization.

Patient Instruction Drives:

Patient instruction is an incredible asset for beating opposition and cultivating acknowledgment of all encompassing methodologies. Clinics can foster patient instruction drives that give data about the advantages, wellbeing, and proof supporting integral treatments. Enabling patients with information improves their comprehension and supports dynamic cooperation in all encompassing consideration plans.

Research Drives in All encompassing Recuperating:

Leading and advancing exploration in all encompassing mending adds to building a strong proof base. Medical services foundations can lay out research drives that investigate the viability and wellbeing of corresponding treatments, patient results, and the general effect of all encompassing methodologies. Research discoveries reinforce the validity of all encompassing recuperating and give important bits of knowledge to both medical care experts and the more extensive academic local area.

7.1 Addressing Skepticism and Resistance

Tending to Suspicion and Opposition: Building a Scaffold Between Comprehensive Recuperating and Ordinary Medication in Multispeciality Emergency clinics

The reconciliation of comprehensive recuperating into the domain of multispeciality emergency clinics is met with wariness and opposition, established in the verifiable strength of proof based rehearses and the customary clinical model. Tending to these difficulties requires a smart methodology that recognizes the worries, dissipates confusions, and constructs a scaffold between comprehensive recuperating and ordinary medication. This investigation dives into the wellsprings of wariness and opposition and proposes methodologies for cultivating acknowledgment and joint effort chasing after exhaustive patient consideration.

Wellsprings of Suspicion and Obstruction:

Logical Incredulity:

Incredulity frequently emerges from established researchers' interest for thorough proof to help clinical intercessions. The comprehensive mending worldview, which incorporates a great many practices, may not necessarily adjust to conventional clinical preliminary techniques. The absence of deep rooted logical proof for a few corresponding treatments adds to wariness among medical care experts who focus on proof based rehearses.

Social and Institutional Dormancy:

Clinics and medical services organizations are well established in laid out customs and conventions. Presenting all encompassing recuperating difficulties the current social and institutional standards, prompting obstruction. Wariness might come from worries about disturbing laid out rehearses, expected clashes with traditional therapies, and the anxiety toward going amiss from demonstrated clinical conventions.

Absence of Normalization:

The shortfall of normalized rehearses inside comprehensive recuperating adds to wariness. Not at all like traditional medication, which complies to severe conventions and rules, comprehensive methodologies fluctuate generally in their application and viability. The absence of generally acknowledged guidelines raises worries about consistency, wellbeing, and the unwavering quality of all encompassing intercessions.

Misinterpretations and Shame:

Misinterpretations and shame encompassing comprehensive mending further fuel suspicion. Some view corresponding treatments as "elective" as opposed to integrative, seeing them as problematic or even enchanted. The relationship with elective medication rehearses that need logical approval adds to the doubt and hesitance to embrace all encompassing methodologies inside the standard medical care local area.

Restricted Understanding and Training:

Doubt is in many cases established in a restricted comprehension of all encompassing standards and practices. Medical care experts might need openness to comprehensive mending during their conventional training, prompting an information hole. Without complete training on the proof supporting different corresponding treatments and the comprehensive worldview, wariness continues.

Techniques for Tending to Doubt and Opposition:

Building a Proof Base:

To beat logical doubt, there is a need to fabricate a powerful proof base for all encompassing mending rehearses. Directing very much planned research concentrates on that stick to logical systems is fundamental. Joint efforts between all encompassing specialists and analysts can add to the age of top notch proof that upholds the wellbeing and adequacy of correlative treatments.

Foundation of Integrative Medication Divisions:

Making committed integrative medication divisions inside multispeciality emergency clinics gives an organized climate to comprehensive recuperating. These divisions can act as focuses of greatness, cultivating joint effort among ordinary and comprehensive professionals. By exhibiting effective integrative models, clinics can assemble validity and show the substantial advantages of comprehensive methodologies.

Instructive Drives for Medical services Experts:

Tending to restricted understanding and schooling includes carrying out thorough instructive drives for medical services experts. Coordinating comprehensive standards into clinical educational programs, offering proceeding with schooling programs, and giving chances to involved preparing in corresponding treatments add to a more educated and liberal medical services labor force.

Advancing Interdisciplinary Joint effort:

Encouraging coordinated effort between medical services experts from different disciplines is significant for beating opposition. Multidisciplinary gatherings, case conversations, and joint preparation programs set out open doors for ordinary and comprehensive experts to share bits of knowledge, dissipate legends, and gain from one another. Interdisciplinary cooperation improves shared regard and understanding.

Clear Correspondence of Advantages and Dangers:

Straightforward correspondence about the advantages and dangers of comprehensive mending rehearses is fundamental for scattering misguided judgments. Giving clear data about proof based reciprocal treatments, their likely combination with ordinary medicines, and the positive effect on persistent results helps construct trust and decreases wariness.

Advancement of Clinical Rules:

To address worries about the absence of normalization, medical services establishments can team up with comprehensive experts to foster proof based clinical rules for correlative treatments. These rules guarantee consistency by and by, improve patient security, and give a system to the mindful joining of comprehensive methodologies into traditional clinical consideration.

Patient-Focused Approach:

Embracing a patient-focused approach is significant in building acknowledgment for comprehensive mending. Medical care experts ought to focus on grasping patients' inclinations, convictions, and social foundations. By effectively including patients in direction, fitting treatment plans to individual necessities, and regarding their decisions, medical services suppliers can establish a strong climate that values all encompassing standards.

Research Scattering and Public Mindfulness:

Scattering research discoveries and raising public mindfulness about all encompassing recuperating add to separating confusions and disgrace. State funded schooling efforts, instructive materials, and local area occasions assist with demystifying all encompassing practices and feature the proof supporting their joining into ordinary medical care.

Authority Backing and Promotion:

Solid authority backing and promotion are fundamental for defeating institutional latency. Emergency clinic overseers and pioneers assume an essential part in supporting the coordination of all encompassing mending. By upholding for assets, establishing a steady climate, and adjusting hierarchical objectives to comprehensive standards, pioneers can work with a culture shift inside medical services organizations.

Continuous Coordination with Clear Conventions:

To address fears of disturbing laid out rehearses, a slow and staged reconciliation of all encompassing mending with clear conventions is suggested. Experimental runs programs, at first centered around unambiguous divisions or patient populaces, take into consideration cautious checking, assessment, and change of all encompassing methodologies inside a controlled climate before more extensive execution.

Patient Tributes and Examples of overcoming adversity:

Sharing patient tributes and examples of overcoming adversity can be an integral asset in defeating wariness. Genuine encounters of people who have profited from all encompassing methodologies act as convincing accounts that resound with both medical services experts and the general population. These accounts adapt comprehensive mending, accentuating its effect on individual prosperity.

7.2 Training Healthcare Professionals for Holistic Care

Preparing Medical care Experts for All encompassing Consideration: Overcoming any issues Between Traditional Medication and Comprehensive Recuperating in Multispeciality Clinics

The fruitful mix of all encompassing mending into multispeciality medical clinics relies on the compelling preparation of medical services experts. As the medical services scene develops, there is a developing acknowledgment of the need to furnish experts with the information, abilities, and mentalities important to give all encompassing consideration. This investigation dives into the difficulties related with preparing medical care experts for all encompassing consideration and proposes complete techniques to overcome any issues between traditional medication and comprehensive recuperating.

Challenges in Preparing Medical services Experts for Comprehensive Consideration:

Restricted Openness and Instruction:

Numerous medical care experts get restricted openness to comprehensive standards and works on during their conventional training. The customary clinical educational program frequently underlines proof based rehearses and clinical abilities, generally ruling out the investigation of all encompassing methodologies. This restricted openness brings about an information hole and an absence of knowledge of the different scope of comprehensive recuperating modalities.

Distrust and Obstruction:

Distrust and obstruction among medical services experts present huge difficulties to comprehensive consideration preparing. Profoundly instilled social standards inside the clinical local area, combined with distrust about the logical legitimacy of specific corresponding treatments, can upset the acknowledgment of comprehensive standards. Defeating this opposition requires custom-made instructive systems that address assumptions and misguided judgments.

Time Requirements in Medical care Settings:

The requesting idea of medical services settings, described by occupied timetables and high tolerant burdens, presents a test for integrating all encompassing consideration preparing. Medical care experts might see time limitations as a hindrance to taking part in extra preparation programs. Incorporating all encompassing preparation flawlessly into existing instructive structures becomes fundamental to oblige these time imperatives.

Need for Interdisciplinary Cooperation:

All encompassing consideration frequently includes interdisciplinary cooperation, requiring medical care experts to work flawlessly across different fortes. In any case, conventional clinical training will in general be siloed, with restricted accentuation on cooperative abilities. Overcoming any issues among disciplines and cultivating compelling correspondence among medical services experts are basic parts of all encompassing consideration preparing.

Incorporation with Regular Clinical Conventions:

The test lies in coordinating all encompassing consideration preparing with regular clinical conventions. Medical services experts might be worried about likely contentions among comprehensive and proof based rehearses. Adjusting all encompassing consideration to laid out clinical conventions and guaranteeing that it supplements as opposed to goes against regular medicines requires cautious route.

Techniques for Complete Preparation in All encompassing Consideration:

Curricular Mix and Development:

To address the restricted openness in conventional clinical schooling, a key technique is the curricular reconciliation and development of all encompassing consideration parts. Clinical schools and preparing projects can incorporate modules on all encompassing standards, integral treatments, and patient-focused care into existing educational programs. This extension guarantees that future medical services experts get more thorough training that incorporates both regular and comprehensive viewpoints.

Proceeding with Schooling Projects:

Offering proceeding with instruction programs custom-made to medical services experts at different profession stages is fundamental for connecting the information hole. These projects can give inside and out preparing on unambiguous comprehensive modalities, care practices, and patient relational abilities. By making proceeding with instruction open and pertinent, medical care experts can keep up to date with arising comprehensive methodologies and standards.

Experiential Learning Potential open doors:

Active experiential learning is an integral asset in comprehensive consideration preparing. Medical services experts can profit from vivid encounters like studios, reenactments, and patient communications that open them to the pragmatic utilization of comprehensive standards. Experiential learning cultivates a more profound comprehension and appreciation for the all encompassing way to deal with patient consideration.

Developing a Culture of Receptiveness:

Beating incredulity and opposition requires a social shift inside medical services organizations. Preparing projects ought to underscore the development of receptiveness and an eagerness to investigate different recuperating modalities. Making a culture that esteems the reconciliation of comprehensive consideration adds to a more responsive and cooperative medical care climate.

Interdisciplinary Preparation Drives:

Tending to the requirement for interdisciplinary joint effort includes planning preparing drives that unite experts from different medical care disciplines. Cooperative studios, case-based learning, and shared preparing encounters empower medical services suppliers to see the value in one another's viewpoints, convey really, and work solidly toward all encompassing patient consideration.

Joining of Comprehensive Consideration into Recreation Preparing:

Reproduction preparing, usually used to improve clinical abilities, can be reached out to integrate situations that include comprehensive consideration. This approach permits medical care experts to work on coordinating all encompassing standards into patient communications in a controlled climate. Mimicked situations can cover correspondence systems, comprehensive appraisals, and the fuse of integral treatments.

Mentorship and Friend Backing Projects:

Laying out mentorship projects and companion encouraging groups of people cultivates a strong learning climate for medical services experts taking part in all encompassing consideration preparing. Experienced tutors can direct amateurs through the difficulties of consolidating all encompassing methodologies, share bits of knowledge, and offer continuous help. Peer encouraging groups of people work with cooperative learning and the trading of best practices.

Customized Preparing for Explicit Claims to fame:

Perceiving the variety of medical services claims to fame, preparing projects ought to be custom-made to the particular requirements of various disciplines. For instance, preparing for attendants might zero in on comprehensive nursing rehearses, while preparing for doctors might dig into integrative medication. Fitting preparation to the remarkable necessities of every specialty guarantees importance and relevance.

Clear Correspondence of Proof and Exploration:

Tending to suspicion among medical care experts requires clear correspondence of the proof supporting all encompassing practices. Preparing projects ought to underline the current collection of exploration on corresponding treatments, care rehearses, and comprehensive methodologies. Introducing logical proof forms certainty and validity, assisting medical services experts with understanding the reasoning for consolidating all encompassing consideration.

Joining of Comprehensive Consideration in Proficient Improvement Plans:

Empowering medical services experts to remember comprehensive consideration for their expert advancement plans builds up the significance of continuous learning. Establishments can uphold this by perceiving and compensating experts who take part in comprehensive consideration preparing, go to important meetings, and add to the joining of all encompassing standards inside their training.

Coordinated effort with All encompassing Professionals:

Working together with experienced all encompassing professionals enhances preparing programs by giving certifiable bits of knowledge and points of view. All encompassing specialists can share their ability, guide medical services experts in figuring out the comprehensive worldview, and add to the advancement of preparing educational plans that mirror the all encompassing way to deal with care.

Advancement of Taking care of oneself Practices for Medical services Experts:

All encompassing consideration preparing shouldn't just zero in on quiet consideration yet additionally on the prosperity of medical care experts themselves. Consolidating taking care of oneself practices, stress the executives methods, and care preparing into comprehensive consideration programs upholds the psychological, close to home, and actual prosperity of medical services suppliers.

7.3 Overcoming Financial and Operational Challenges

Beating Monetary and Functional Difficulties in Coordinating All encompassing Recuperating into Multispeciality Clinics

The reconciliation of all encompassing recuperating into multispeciality clinics brings groundbreaking potential for patient consideration however isn't without monetary and functional difficulties. As medical services establishments explore this intricate scene, they experience impediments connected with asset designation, monetary manageability, and functional changes. This investigation digs into the monetary and functional difficulties related with the reconciliation of all encompassing mending and proposes systems to defeat these obstacles, encouraging an agreeable mix of customary and comprehensive consideration inside multispeciality clinic settings.

Monetary Difficulties:

Asset Distribution and Financial plan Requirements:

Coordinating comprehensive mending frequently requires a redistribution of assets, including financing for preparing programs, recruiting all encompassing specialists, and making committed spaces for comprehensive consideration. Clinic financial plans are ordinarily close, and getting extra assets for all encompassing drives can challenge. The apparent monetary strain might prompt opposition from medical clinic chairmen and partners.

Techniques:

Money saving advantage Examination: Lead an exhaustive money saving advantage investigation to show the drawn out monetary advantages of all encompassing mending, like superior patient results, expanded patient fulfillment, and possible expense reserve funds in specific regions.

Award Amazing open doors: Investigate award potential open doors and associations with establishments that help integrative and comprehensive medical services drives. Outer subsidizing can offer the fundamental monetary help to launch and support all encompassing projects.

Repayment Difficulties for Comprehensive Administrations:

All encompassing administrations frequently fall outside the traditional repayment structures, representing a monetary test for emergency clinics. Protection suppliers may not cover specific corresponding treatments, making a difference between the apparent worth of all encompassing administrations and their monetary suitability inside the ongoing medical services repayment model.

Techniques:

Support for Repayment Changes: Backer for changes in repayment strategies to incorporate all encompassing administrations. Team up with industry associations, policymakers, and protection suppliers to exhibit the worth of all encompassing consideration and present a defense for extended repayment inclusion.

Advancement of Cross breed Installment Models: Investigate the improvement of mixture installment models that integrate both traditional and comprehensive administrations. This approach can guarantee monetary manageability while lining up with advancing models of patient-focused and esteem based care.

Staffing Expenses and Preparing Costs:

Recruiting and preparing all encompassing professionals, as well as instructing existing staff on comprehensive standards, cause extra staffing expenses and preparing costs. Clinics might be worried about the monetary ramifications of putting resources into specific preparation projects and coordinating new staff individuals with mastery in all encompassing methodologies.

Procedures:

Cooperative Preparation Projects: Team up with outside all encompassing preparation programs and instructive establishments to share the expense and assets for staff preparing. Joint drives can give practical arrangements while guaranteeing that medical services experts get exhaustive and normalized preparing.

Broadly educating Projects: Execute broadly educating programs that permit existing staff to obtain essential information and abilities in all encompassing consideration. This approach limits the requirement for extra employing as well as advances a cooperative and interdisciplinary medical care climate.

Functional Difficulties:

Protection from Social Shift:

Coordinating all encompassing mending requires a social shift inside the clinic climate. Opposition from medical services experts familiar with regular practices might impede the consistent reception of comprehensive methodologies. Opposition can appear in distrust, hesitance to change, and difficulties in laying out a strong social structure that embraces both regular and comprehensive consideration.

Techniques:

Authority Backing and Correspondence: Gain solid administration support for the social shift toward comprehensive consideration. Successful correspondence from medical clinic administration about the vision, benefits, and long haul objectives of all encompassing coordination is pivotal in conquering obstruction and cultivating a common perspective among staff.

Experimental runs Projects: Start test cases programs in unambiguous divisions or units to show the advantages of comprehensive consideration in a controlled climate. Examples of overcoming adversity from these pilot drives can act as strong impetuses for beating obstruction and collecting support from medical services experts.

Functional Work process Mix:

Incorporating all encompassing consideration into existing functional work processes presents difficulties connected with patient booking, documentation, and co-ordinated effort among various claims to fame. Emergency clinics should explore the intricacies of integrating all encompassing appraisals and mediations flawlessly into customary clinical work processes without disturbing laid out conventions.

Techniques:

Interdisciplinary Consideration Groups: Lay out interdisciplinary consideration groups that incorporate both customary and all encompassing professionals. Cultivate cooperation and open correspondence among colleagues to guarantee a durable way to deal with patient consideration. This approach works with the incorporation of all encompassing evaluations and mediations inside existing work processes.

Use of Wellbeing Data Innovation: Influence wellbeing data innovation to smooth out functional cycles. Execute electronic wellbeing record (EHR) frameworks that consider consistent documentation of all encompassing appraisals and mediations. Reconciliation with EHR frameworks guarantees that all encompassing consideration turns into a basic piece of patient records.

Space and Foundation Necessities:

Making devoted spaces for all encompassing consideration, for example, contemplation rooms or integrative consideration habitats, may require actual space and framework changes. Emergency clinics might confront difficulties in reusing existing spaces or distributing assets for new development, particularly when space is along with some hidden costs.

Systems:

Versatile Utilization of Existing Spaces: Amplify the versatile utilization of existing spaces to oblige comprehensive consideration administrations. Convert underutilized regions into all encompassing consideration spaces or assign adaptable spaces that can fill both regular and comprehensive needs.

Coordinated effort with Offices The executives: Team up intimately with offices the board to investigate practical answers for framework changes. Inventive critical thinking and imaginative plan ideas can assist with improving space without compromising the medical clinic's general usefulness.

Patient Schooling and Commitment:

All encompassing consideration frequently requires dynamic patient commitment and instruction, which can strain functional assets. Medical clinics should track down proficient ways of teaching patients about all encompassing standards, include them in shared direction, and support dynamic cooperation in their comprehensive consideration plans.

Procedures:

Advanced Wellbeing Stages: Use computerized wellbeing stages, like patient gateways and portable applications, to convey instructive materials and connect with patients in their comprehensive consideration. These stages give a helpful and versatile method for arriving at patients while limiting the burden on functional assets.

Patient Pilots and Backing Projects: Carry out quiet guide projects or backing drives that guide patients through their all encompassing consideration venture. Committed work force can give customized help, answer questions, and work with correspondence among patients and medical care suppliers, improving the general patient experience.

Assessment of All encompassing Results:

Estimating the effect of all encompassing consideration on understanding results presents functional difficulties. Medical clinics need powerful assessment measurements and frameworks to evaluate the viability of comprehensive mediations, patient fulfillment, and the general mix of all encompassing methodologies into the medical services conveyance model.

Techniques:

Execution of Result Measures: Characterize and carry out result estimates that line up with the objectives of comprehensive consideration. These actions might incorporate patient-revealed results, enhancements in personal satisfaction, decrease in feelings of anxiety, and generally speaking patient fulfillment. Routinely survey and investigate these results to show the worth of comprehensive consideration.

Joint effort with Exploration Foundations: Team up with research organizations to direct examinations on the effect of all encompassing consideration inside medical clinic settings. Taking part in research drives adds to the proof base as well as gives significant experiences into functional changes and regions for development.

Quality Confirmation and Normalization:

Guaranteeing the quality and normalization of comprehensive consideration rehearses presents functional difficulties. Medical clinics should lay out clear rules, conventions, and quality confirmation systems to keep up with consistency in the conveyance of comprehensive administrations across various divisions and claims to fame.

Systems:

Improvement of Comprehensive Consideration Boards: Structure all encompassing consideration councils inside the medical clinic design to direct the normalization of practices. These councils can incorporate delegates from different strengths and disciplines, working cooperatively to lay out rules, survey conventions, and guarantee quality affirmation in all encompassing consideration.

Nonstop Preparation and Expert Turn of events: Execute ceaseless preparation and expert improvement programs for medical services experts associated with comprehensive consideration. These projects guarantee that specialists stay refreshed on advancing norms, proof based practices, and quality affirmation measures.

Chapter 8

Future Trends in Multispeciality Hospital Excellence

The scene of multispeciality clinics is ceaselessly developing, driven by headways in clinical science, mechanical advancement, moving patient assumptions, and a developing accentuation on comprehensive and patient-focused care. Expecting future patterns in multispeciality medical clinic greatness is basic for medical services establishments to adjust, flourish, and keep conveying top caliber, exhaustive medical care administrations. This investigation dives into a few key future patterns that are ready to shape the scene of multispeciality clinics.

Incorporation of Man-made consciousness (computer based intelligence) and Innovation:

The incorporation of man-made consciousness (simulated intelligence) and cutting edge innovations is a groundbreaking pattern that holds gigantic potential for multispeciality emergency clinics. Artificial intelligence applications, for example, AI calculations and prescient investigation, can improve analytic exactness, upgrade treatment designs, and smooth out managerial cycles. Mechanical technology and telemedicine are additionally expected to assume critical parts, empowering far off counsels, careful intercessions, and patient observing. The consistent joining of these innovations won't just further develop proficiency yet additionally raise the general patient experience.

Customized and Accuracy Medication:

The eventual fate of multispeciality clinic greatness lies in the domain of customized and accuracy medication. Progresses in genomics, sub-atomic profiling, and biomarker research are making ready for customized treatment draws near. Emergency clinics will progressively use hereditary and atomic information to redo treatment plans in view of a singular's extraordinary hereditary cosmetics and sickness profile. This shift towards accuracy medication holds the commitment of further developed treatment results, diminished secondary effects, and a more designated way to deal with patient consideration.

All encompassing and Integrative Medical services Models:

The pattern towards all encompassing and integrative medical care models is picking up speed, underscoring a far reaching approach that tends to actual infirmities as well as mental, profound, and social prosperity. Multispeciality clinics are supposed to coordinate reciprocal treatments, care rehearses, and comprehensive consideration standards into their administration contributions. This comprehensive methodology recognizes the interconnected idea of wellbeing and expects to furnish patients with an all the more balanced and customized medical care insight.

Accentuation on Preventive Medical services:

The fate of multispeciality clinic greatness will see a critical shift towards preventive medical care. Emergency clinics will progressively zero in on proactive measures, wellbeing screenings, and way of life mediations to forestall the beginning of illnesses. Populace wellbeing the board procedures will assume a vital part in distinguishing in danger populaces and carrying out designated mediations to advance generally speaking wellbeing and prosperity.

Patient-Driven and Experience-Driven Care:

Patient-centricity will keep on being a main thrust in forming multispeciality medical clinic greatness. The future pattern stresses upgrading the general patient experience, from the second a patient enters the medical clinic to post-release care. This incorporates customized treatment plans, straightforward correspondence, and an emphasis on tolerant fulfillment. Emergency clinics will put resources into establishing mending conditions that focus on the profound and mental prosperity of patients.

Interconnected Medical care Biological systems:

The eventual fate of multispeciality emergency clinics lies in the formation of interconnected medical services biological systems. Cooperative associations between emergency clinics, essential consideration suppliers, subject matter experts, and local area based associations will turn out to be progressively common. Consistent information sharing, interoperability of wellbeing records, and composed care conveyance will guarantee a continuum of care that rises above conventional storehouses, prompting more proficient and powerful medical care administrations.

Far off Understanding Observing and Home Medical care:

Propels in innovation, combined with the developing accentuation on persistent driven care, will drive the pattern towards far off understanding checking and home medical services. Wearable gadgets, telehealth stages, and remote checking devices will empower medical care suppliers to follow patients' wellbeing continuously, considering early mediation and diminishing the requirement for clinic visits. Home medical care administrations will grow, furnishing patients with the accommodation of getting clinical consideration in the solace of their homes.

Center around Psychological wellness and Prosperity:

The eventual fate of multispeciality emergency clinic greatness perceives the essential job of psychological wellness in by and large prosperity. Medical clinics will progressively focus on emotional well-being administrations, incorporating mental consideration, advising, and health programs into their contributions. The disgrace encompassing psychological well-being will keep on lessening, cultivating a climate where patients feel happy with looking for and getting psychological wellness support close by customary clinical consideration.

Natural Supportability Drives:

Manageability is arising as a critical pattern in multispeciality clinic greatness. Clinics are perceiving the natural effect of medical services rehearses and are making strides towards eco-accommodating and reasonable drives. From energy-productive foundation to squander decrease and ecologically cognizant store network the executives, emergency clinics are lining up with more extensive cultural objectives of manageability and corporate social obligation.

Information Security and Online protection Measures:

With the rising dependence on computerized advances and the huge measures of delicate patient information produced, information security and network protection estimates will be vital. Multispeciality emergency clinics will put resources into strong network safety structures to safeguard patient data, guarantee the respectability of clinical records, and shield against potential digital dangers. This incorporates executing progressed encryption techniques, standard security reviews, and staff preparing on network safety best practices.

Worldwide Wellbeing Cooperation and Pandemic Readiness:

The worldwide interconnectedness of medical care frameworks has been highlighted by late pandemics. Multispeciality clinics are supposed to take part in expanded cooperation on a worldwide scale to share information, assets, and best practices. Pandemic readiness plans will be basic to emergency clinic activities, guaranteeing quick and viable reactions to arising general wellbeing emergencies.

8.1 Technological Advancements in Holistic Healthcare

Mechanical Progressions in All encompassing Medical services: Spearheading the Fate of Thorough Prosperity

The crossing point of innovation and medical care has introduced another time of potential outcomes, upsetting the manner in which we approach comprehensive medical care. As society turns out to be progressively interconnected and carefully determined, creative advancements are assuming a crucial part in upgrading comprehensive practices, customized care, and by and large prosperity. This investigation digs into the innovative progressions forming the scene of all encompassing medical services and their significant effect on the conveyance of far reaching patient-focused care.

Computerized reasoning (simulated intelligence) and AI:

Computerized reasoning (man-made intelligence) and AI are at the bleeding edge of mechanical headways in all encompassing medical services. These advancements have the ability to examine tremendous measures of information, distinguish designs, and create experiences that can illuminate customized treatment plans. In comprehensive consideration, man-made intelligence is being used to survey way of life factors, break down quiet ways of behaving, and tailor mediations to individual requirements. AI calculations can anticipate wellbeing gambles, empowering proactive and preventive measures to improve generally prosperity.

Computer generated Reality (VR) and Increased Reality (AR):

Computer generated Reality (VR) and Increased Reality (AR) are changing the scene of all encompassing medical care by giving vivid and intelligent encounters. In restorative settings, VR is being utilized for directed contemplation, stress decrease, and openness treatment. AR applications improve the patient's actual climate, over-laying computerized data onto this present reality. These advances make drawing in and remedial encounters that add to mental, close to home, and profound prosperity.

Telehealth and Distant Patient Observing:

The ascent of telehealth and distant patient checking has become especially articu-lated in all encompassing medical services. Telehealth stages empower patients to get to all encompassing professionals from a distance, encouraging coherence of care without geological requirements. Moreover, far off tolerant checking gadgets, like wearables and shrewd sensors, consider continuous following of essential signs, active work, and other wellbeing measurements. This innovation upgrades all encompassing consider-ation by empowering professionals to screen patients in their regular surroundings, advancing a more extensive comprehension of their prosperity.

Wellbeing Applications and Wearable Innovation:

The expansion of wellbeing applications and wearable innovation is enabling people to effectively participate in their comprehensive prosperity. These applications give devices to following active work, checking rest designs, rehearsing care, and overseeing pressure. Wearable gadgets, like wellness trackers and smartwatches, offer continuous input on different wellbeing measurements. Coordinating comprehensive standards, these innovations urge people to make proactive strides towards keeping a reasonable and solid way of life.

Genomic Medication and Customized Therapeutics:

Headways in genomic medication have introduced another time of customized therapeutics in comprehensive medical care. Hereditary testing can give bits of knowledge into a singular's inclination to specific ailments, permitting specialists to tailor comprehensive intercessions in light of hereditary variables. This customized approach guarantees that treatment plans line up with a patient's special hereditary cosmetics, improving the viability of comprehensive treatments and limiting possible unfavorable impacts.

Blockchain for Wellbeing Information Security:

The utilization of blockchain innovation is addressing concerns connected with wellbeing information security and protection in all encompassing medical services. Blockchain guarantees secure and alter safe capacity of wellbeing records, encouraging trust among patients and specialists. Patients have more prominent command over their wellbeing information, permitting them to impart explicit data to all encompass-ing professionals while keeping up with privacy. This decentralized and secure way to deal with wellbeing information the board upgrades straightforwardness and the respectability of patient data.

Shrewd Sensors and Web of Things (IoT):

Shrewd sensors and the Web of Things (IoT) are instrumental in all encompassing medical services by giving constant information to customized mediations. Wearable shrewd sensors can screen physiological boundaries, natural factors, and, surprisingly, profound states. This information is then coordinated into all encompassing consideration plans, empowering professionals to present ideal and custom-made suggestions. The IoT works with consistent correspondence between gadgets, making an organization that improves the general checking and the board of patients' all encompassing prosperity.

Biometric Criticism and Biofeedback Gadgets:

Biometric criticism and biofeedback gadgets offer people experiences into their physiological reactions and empower them to effectively take part in their prosperity. These gadgets measure boundaries, for example, pulse inconstancy, skin conductance, and muscle pressure, giving constant input on the body's pressure reactions. Experts in all encompassing medical care utilize this data to direct patients in care rehearses, stress decrease methods, and different mediations pointed toward encouraging comprehensive prosperity.

3D Printing for Customized Prosthetics and Orthotics:

3D printing innovation is altering the field of customized prosthetics and orthotics. In all encompassing medical care, this progression guarantees that people with actual impediments approach tweaked arrangements that line up with their novel requirements. Whether it's a custom orthotic gadget for act support or a prosthetic append-age custom-made to a singular's life structures, 3D printing empowers professionals to give comprehensive arrangements that upgrade both actual capability and in general prosperity.

Normal Language Handling (NLP) for All encompassing Conversational Points of interaction:

Normal Language Handling (NLP) is improving the patient-professional cooperation in all encompassing medical care through conversational connection points. Remote helpers and chatbots furnished with NLP capacities permit patients to take part in normal, language-driven discussions about their prosperity. These connection points give data, direction on all encompassing practices, and basic reassurance, making a more open and intuitive road for people to investigate and upgrade their comprehensive wellbeing.

Mechanical Help with Restoration and Old Consideration:

Advanced mechanics is taking huge steps in giving help with recovery and old consideration inside the comprehensive medical services structure. Mechanical gadgets are intended to help people in recapturing actual capability, giving friendship, and helping with exercises of day to day living. Coordinating these advances into all encompassing consideration guarantees a far reaching way to deal with physical and close to home prosperity, particularly in populaces requiring recovery or older people looking for comprehensive help.

8.2 Emerging Holistic Healing Modalities

Arising All encompassing Mending Modalities: Exploring the Outskirts of Thorough Prosperity

All encompassing mending, established in the way of thinking of tending to the interconnected parts of a singular's wellbeing — physical, mental, close to home, and profound — is seeing a unique development with the rise of creative modalities. As how we might interpret comprehensive prosperity extends, specialists and people the same are investigating and embracing new methodologies that go past customary practices. This investigation dives into the wilderness of arising all encompassing recuperating modalities, featuring their standards, applications, and possible effect on extensive wellbeing.

Hallucinogenic Helped Treatment:

Hallucinogenic helped treatment is earning respect as a groundbreaking methodology for psychological well-being and close to home recuperating. Substances like psilocybin (tracked down in specific mushrooms) and MDMA (usually known as joy) are being explored for their true capacity in dealing with conditions like despondency, nervousness, and post-horrendous pressure problem (PTSD). These substances, when directed in a controlled restorative setting, can prompt modified conditions of cognizance, advancing contemplation, profound delivery, and otherworldly experiences. Advocates contend that hallucinogenic helped treatment can possibly resolve firmly established intense subject matters and add to comprehensive recuperating by cultivating a significant association between the psyche, feelings, and soul.

Sound Recuperating and Vibrational Medication:

Sound mending and vibrational medication tap into the remedial force of sound frequencies to reestablish harmony and advance prosperity. Modalities like sound showers, gong treatment, and Tibetan singing bowl meetings include presenting people to explicit frequencies that resound with various parts of the body and brain. The vibrations are accepted to significantly affect cells, tissues, and energy frameworks, advancing unwinding, stress decrease, and, surprisingly, cell recuperating. Sound mending is progressively incorporated into all encompassing practices as a painless and open method for improving mental and close to home states.

Energy Medication and Biofield Treatments:

Energy medication envelops a different scope of modalities that perceive the job of unpretentious energy fields in advancing wellbeing and mending. Practices like Reiki, needle therapy, and Qi Gong work on the reason that the body has a fiery diagram that impacts physical, mental, and close to home prosperity. Specialists work to adjust and advance the progression of energy through the body, tending to irregular characteristics and supporting the body's regular mending processes. These biofield treatments are acquiring acknowledgment as reciprocal ways to deal with regular clinical mediations, adding to a comprehensive comprehension of wellbeing.

Timberland Washing and Nature Treatment:

Timberland washing, or shinrin-yoku, is a training established in the remedial advantages of submerging oneself in nature. Beginning in Japan, this methodology includes careful and purposeful commitment with common habitats, advancing unwinding, stress decrease, and a feeling of association with the regular world. Research demonstrates that investing energy in nature can decidedly affect psychological wellness, resistant capability, and generally prosperity. Nature treatment extends the extent of comprehensive mending by perceiving the significant impact of the climate on a person's physiological and mental states.

Equine-Helped Treatment:

Equine-helped treatment includes cooperations with ponies to advance close to home development, mindfulness, and relational abilities. This methodology perceives the novel characteristics of ponies, like their awareness and non-critical nature, as impetuses for mending. People take part in exercises like preparing, driving, and riding ponies under the direction of prepared specialists. The dynamic among people and ponies is accepted to reflect relational connections, offering experiences into correspondence styles and close to home examples. Equine-helped treatment adds a dynamic and experiential aspect to comprehensive mending, especially in the domain of close to home and social prosperity.

Weed and Cannabinoid Treatments:

The remedial utilization of weed and cannabinoids is arising as an all encompassing way to deal with address different ailments, including constant torment, nervousness, and sleep deprivation. Cannabinoids, for example, cannabidiol (CBD) and tetrahydrocannabinol (THC), associate with the endocannabinoid framework in the body, impacting processes connected with torment discernment, state of mind, and safe capability. Comprehensive specialists are investigating the capability of pot based treatments to supplement different modalities and improve generally prosperity. In any case, it is vital to take note of that the administrative scene and logical comprehension of weed treatments keep on advancing.

Ayurvedic and Integrative Nourishment:

Ayurveda, the old arrangement of medication from India, is acquiring conspicuousness as a comprehensive recuperating methodology that incorporates nourishment and way of life rehearses. Ayurvedic nourishment underscores the significance of individualized dietary decisions in view of one's dosha, or special protected type. Integrative nourishment joins Ayurvedic standards with present day dietary science, perceiving the effect of food on physical, mental, and close to home wellbeing. By fitting dietary suggestions to a singular's constitution and uneven characters, Ayurvedic and integrative sustenance add to an all encompassing way to deal with supporting the body and brain.

Careful Development Practices:

Careful development rehearses, like Feldenkrais, Alexander Procedure, and careful yoga, center around improving familiarity with body development and arrangement.

These practices underscore the association between development examples, stance, and in general prosperity. By developing care during development, people can foster an elevated feeling of body mindfulness, discharge strain, and work on actual capability. Careful development rehearses add to the all encompassing mending worldview by cultivating a careful and encapsulated way to deal with actual wellbeing.

Integrative Breathwork:

Breathwork modalities, like Holotropic Breathwork and Groundbreaking Breath, investigate the extraordinary force of cognizant and deliberate relaxing. These practices include explicit breathing procedures to initiate modified conditions of cognizance, discharge profound blockages, and advance a feeling of otherworldly association. Integrative breathwork is progressively incorporated into comprehensive mending draws near, perceiving the significant effect of breath on the sensory system, close to home states, and generally speaking imperativeness.

Expressive Expressions Treatments:

Expressive expressions treatments, including workmanship treatment, music treatment, and dance/development treatment, influence the innovative approach to improve close to home articulation and prosperity. These modalities perceive the remedial capability of creative articulation in tending to mental and personal difficulties. Incorporating human expressions into all encompassing recuperating furnishes people with elective roads for self-disclosure, profound delivery, and the development of a comprehensive identity.

8.3 The Role of Research and Innovation in Multispeciality Hospitals

The Job of Exploration and Development in Multispeciality Emergency clinics: Spearheading Advances for Thorough Patient Consideration

Examination and development stand as the foundations of progress in multispeciality emergency clinics, driving groundbreaking advances that shape the scene of patient consideration. In the unique domain of medical care, the reconciliation of state of the art research and creative advances inside multispeciality emergency clinics is instrumental in upgrading demonstrative abilities, therapy modalities, and generally tolerant results. This investigation dives into the crucial job of examination and development in multispeciality clinics and their significant effect on propelling complete and patient-focused care.

1. Accuracy Medication and Customized Treatment Approaches:

    Exploration and development have moved the advancement of accuracy medication, a methodology that tailors clinical treatment to the singular qualities of every patient. Multispeciality emergency clinics are at the front of integrating accuracy medication into their works on, utilizing hereditary data, sub-atomic profiling, and high level demonstrative apparatuses to distinguish explicit biomarkers and alter treatment plans. This individualized methodology considers designated treatments, limiting unfavorable impacts and enhancing treatment viability. Research-driven drives in genomics, proteomics, and different fields add to the continuous improvement of accuracy medication conventions, situating multispeciality emergency clinics as center points for customized and state of the art care.

2. High level Imaging and Demonstrative Advances:
Multispeciality emergency clinics constantly put resources into exploration and development to upgrade indicative imaging advances. From high-goal X-ray and CT sweeps to sub-atomic imaging and positron emanation tomography (PET), these progressions furnish clinicians with definite experiences into the physiological and physical parts of patients. Early discovery of sicknesses, exact conclusion, and ongoing observing of therapy reactions are made conceivable through these imaginative imaging modalities. As exploration in clinical imaging advances, multispeciality clinics rush to embrace cutting edge innovations, cultivating a symptomatic climate that is both exact and complete.

3. Integrative Advancements in Medical procedure and Mediations:
Careful and interventional methodology have gone through extraordinary changes with the joining of creative advances. Research-driven drives in advanced mechanics, negligibly obtrusive procedures, and picture directed mediations have reclassified the scene of careful accuracy and patient recuperation. Multispeciality emergency clinics take part in continuous exploration to assess the wellbeing and adequacy of these innovations, adding to the refinement and reception of cutting edge surgeries. The reconciliation of mechanical technology, increased reality, and telepresence advancements empowers specialists to carry out complex strategies with upgraded accuracy, lessening recuperation times and working on generally quiet results.

4. Telemedicine and Virtual Medical care Stages:
Research in telemedicine and virtual medical care stages has acquired noticeable quality, particularly considering worldwide difficulties like the Coronavirus pandemic. Multispeciality clinics influence telehealth advancements to give far off interviews, screen persistent circumstances, and convey specific consideration to patients independent of geological limitations. Progressing research in the adequacy, availability, and patient fulfillment related with telemedicine adds to the refinement and development of virtual medical care administrations inside multispeciality settings. These stages upgrade patient admittance to multispeciality ability, smooth out care conveyance, and further develop in general medical services openness.

5. Interdisciplinary Exploration Joint efforts:
The idea of multispeciality emergency clinics intrinsically advances interdisciplinary coordinated effort, and exploration drives are no exemption. Cooperative endeavors among experts from different clinical disciplines encourage a comprehensive way to deal with complex clinical difficulties. Research projects that range numerous fortes add to a more extensive comprehension of infections, treatment modalities, and patient consideration pathways. Multispeciality

emergency clinics act as center points for cooperative examination, uniting specialists from different fields to resolve complex clinical issues and trailblazer novel ways to deal with care.

6. Information Examination and Man-made reasoning (artificial intelligence): Multispeciality medical clinics are progressively outfitting the force of information examination and simulated intelligence to get significant experiences from huge datasets. Research in these fields empowers the improvement of prescient models, choice emotionally supportive networks, and information driven procedures for patient consideration. Simulated intelligence applications aid early infection location, risk definition, and treatment streamlining. By consolidating AI calculations, multispeciality emergency clinics improve their symptomatic exactness, smooth out functional cycles, and add to the continuous headways in the field of medical care informatics.

7. Patient-Driven Advancements and Commitment:
Research in quiet driven advancements centers around working on the general patient experience and commitment inside multispeciality medical clinics. From the improvement of easy to use versatile applications for arrangement booking to customized wellbeing entryways that engage patients with admittance to their clinical records, continuous exploration tries to upgrade correspondence, accommodation, and dynamic support in medical services choices. Patient-driven developments add to worked on persistent fulfillment as well as cultivate a cooperative and straightforward medical services climate.

8. Drug Disclosure and Remedial Headways:
Multispeciality emergency clinics take part in research attempts that add to the disclosure of novel medications and helpful mediations. Clinical preliminaries and translational exploration drives inside clinic settings assume an essential part in assessing the wellbeing and viability of new medicines. This obligation to explore in drug advancement positions multispeciality clinics as vital participants in propelling clinical treatments, tending to neglected clinical necessities, and working on the norm of care for patients.

9. Populace Wellbeing The executives Procedures:
Multispeciality medical clinics are progressively engaged with research drives zeroed in on populace wellbeing the board. By dissecting populace wellbeing information, recognizing wellbeing differences, and carrying out preventive procedures, emergency clinics add to local area based medical services intercessions. Research-driven populace wellbeing the board intends to upgrade preventive consideration, decrease medical care incongruities, and further develop the general wellbeing results of different patient populaces.

10. Execution of All encompassing and Integrative Practices:

Investigation into comprehensive and integrative medical care rehearses is building up some decent forward movement inside multispeciality clinics. From care based mediations to integrative oncology draws near, continuous examination investigates the adequacy and advantages of reciprocal treatments close by regular clinical medicines. This integrative exploration adds to the advancement of proof based conventions that perceive the interconnected idea of physical, mental, and profound prosperity.

Chapter 9

Conclusion

The scene of medical services has gone through a significant change with the development of multispeciality emergency clinics, driven by a pledge to comprehensive mending, exploration, and development. The excursion we have investigated highlights the interconnected aspects of comprehensive medical services, accentuating the combination of conventional and current medication inside the multidisciplinary structure of multispeciality clinics.

The idea of Comprehensive Recuperating Multispeciality Emergency clinic Greatness epitomizes a dream where patient consideration rises above the traditional limits of clinical claims to fame. It imagines a climate where the physical, mental, close to home, and profound parts of wellbeing combine, cultivating a complete methodology that perceives the many-sided exchange of these aspects in the prosperity of people.

Comprehensive Mending, as clarified in our investigation, envelops a bunch of modalities that stretch out past customary clinical practices. From arising all encompassing recuperating modalities like hallucinogenic helped treatment, sound mending, and nature treatment to laid out practices, for example, Ayurveda and care, the comprehensive methodology recognizes the variety of human encounters and fits care to the one of a kind requirements of every person.

This approach tends to the side effects as well as looks to comprehend and mend the main drivers, adding to a more significant and manageable prosperity.

The meaning of Multispeciality Clinics in this worldview is apparent. These establishments act as focal points where clinical skill from different disciplines combines to give complete and cooperative consideration. The incorporation of examination and development inside multispeciality clinics drives headways that rethink the norm of patient consideration. From accuracy medication and high level imaging advances to telemedicine and computerized reasoning, these emergency clinics are at the front of spearheading drives that upgrade indicative precision, treatment viability, and generally speaking medical services availability.

The Underpinnings of Comprehensive Mending, as investigated, rest upon a profound comprehension of the interconnectedness of brain, body, and soul. This understanding is essential to the all encompassing medical care approach, directing specialists in fitting mediations that address the aggregate of a singular's wellbeing. The verifiable points of view on all encompassing medication uncover that this approach is certainly not a new peculiarity however has establishes in old mending customs that perceived the comprehensive idea of human wellbeing. As present day medication keeps on advancing, the joining of all encompassing standards becomes necessary to accomplishing complete and patient-focused care.

The Development of Multispeciality Emergency clinics and the Coordination of Conventional and Current Medication connote a change in outlook in medical care conveyance. It mirrors an acknowledgment that the blend of different clinical methodologies is fundamental for giving balanced and compelling consideration. The Job of Multispeciality Emergency clinics in All encompassing Mending, as examined, underlines the vital job these foundations play in cultivating cooperation among strengths, guaranteeing complete patient consideration, and embracing the comprehensive recuperating worldview.

Complete Patient Consideration, inside the setting of multispeciality emergency clinics, reaches out past clinical medicines to incorporate the general prosperity of patients. From integrative medication divisions and all encompassing nursing practices to restoration programs and mental prosperity drives, far reaching patient consideration exemplifies a comprehensive methodology that tends to the different requirements of people all through their medical services venture.

Cooperation Among Strengths is a key part in accomplishing the all encompassing medical care vision. The compelling joint effort of experts from assorted fields guarantees that patients get incorporated and composed care. Comprehensive Way to deal with Conclusion and Therapy highlights the significance of thinking about the entire individual in clinical evaluations and mediations.

By perceiving the interconnected idea of physical and psychological well-being, specialists can tailor demonstrative and treatment designs that line up with the comprehensive mending worldview.

Establishing a Mending Climate and Planning Patient-Accommodating Spaces add to the general patient experience inside multispeciality medical clinics. These drives perceive the effect of the actual climate on close to home prosperity and underline the significance of making spaces that advance mending and solace.

Coordinating Elective Treatments and Advancing Mental Prosperity in Medical clinic Settings broaden the range of patient consideration to incorporate corresponding treatments and emotional well-being support. These drives perceive that a comprehensive way to deal with wellbeing incorporates actual infirmities as well as mental and profound states.

All encompassing Mending Practices in Multispeciality Emergency clinics highlight the significance of embracing a comprehensive way of thinking all through the medical care continuum. From integrative medication divisions and all encompassing nursing practices to restoration programs and mental prosperity drives, these practices add to a more complete and patient-focused approach.

Integrative Medication Divisions and Comprehensive Nursing Practices epitomize the obligation to an all encompassing medical services approach. These offices and practices coordinate reciprocal treatments, patient instruction, and comprehensive standards into the standard medical care model, giving patients an all the more balanced and customized insight.

Comprehensive Restoration Projects and Fruitful Execution perceive the significance of all encompassing methodologies in recovery and the requirement for viable systems to carry out comprehensive recuperating standards. These projects add to a more complete and patient-focused restoration experience.

Instances of Multispeciality Clinics Embracing Comprehensive Mending exhibit genuine cases where foundations have effectively coordinated all encompassing standards into their medical services conveyance models. These models act as motivations for others on the excursion toward all encompassing medical care.

Influence on Understanding Results and Fulfillment underscores the beneficial outcomes of comprehensive medical care on tolerant prosperity and fulfillment. By tending to the different requirements of patients and perceiving the interconnected idea of wellbeing, all encompassing methodologies add to further developed results and in general persistent fulfillment.

Illustrations Gained from Genuine Encounters and Difficulties and Arrangements give experiences into the pragmatic parts of executing comprehensive recuperating in multispeciality clinics. These examples feature the significance of addressing moves and tracking down inventive answers for encourage the reconciliation of comprehensive standards into medical care rehearses.

Addressing Distrust and Obstruction perceives that the change to comprehensive medical care might experience suspicion and opposition from different partners. Methodologies for tending to these difficulties include training, correspondence, and a pledge to exhibiting the worth of all encompassing methodologies.

Preparing Medical services Experts for Comprehensive Consideration underscores the significance of planning medical services experts to embrace and incorporate all encompassing standards into their training. Schooling, preparing programs, and persistent expert improvement assume critical parts in guaranteeing that specialists are prepared to convey comprehensive consideration.

Defeating Monetary and Functional Difficulties recognizes the intricacies of incorporating all encompassing recuperating into multispeciality medical clinics and the need to address monetary and functional contemplations. Methodologies incorporate pushing for repayment changes, enhancing functional work processes, and drawing in patients successfully.

Future Patterns in Multispeciality Emergency clinic Greatness expects the direction of medical services by recognizing arising patterns. From the joining of man-made reasoning and customized medication to an emphasis on preventive medical care and worldwide wellbeing joint effort, these patterns shape the future scene of multispeciality clinic greatness.

Mechanical Headways in Comprehensive Medical care investigates the extraordinary effect of innovation on all encompassing mending rehearses. From man-made consciousness and augmented reality to wearable innovation and biofeedback gadgets, mechanical headways improve the conveyance of all encompassing medical care and engage people to effectively participate in their prosperity.

Arising All encompassing Recuperating Modalities wanders into the outskirts of creative ways to deal with prosperity. Hallucinogenic helped treatment, sound mending, energy medication, and expressive expressions treatments represent the variety of modalities that add to the all encompassing recuperating worldview.

The Job of Exploration and Development in Multispeciality Emergency clinics highlights the vital job of examination and advancement in propelling medical care. Accuracy medication, high level imaging advancements, telemedicine, and patient-driven developments are among the key regions where exploration and development drive progress.

9.1 Recap of Holistic Healing in Multispeciality Hospitals

Recap of All encompassing Recuperating in Multispeciality Medical clinics: Exploring the Interconnected Scene of Far reaching Care

As we ponder the complex excursion through the domains of Comprehensive Recuperating in Multispeciality Emergency clinics, it becomes evident that this change in outlook in medical services isn't simply a pattern however a groundbreaking methodology that perceives the many-sided transaction of physical, mental, close to home, and otherworldly aspects in the prosperity of people. This recap looks to distil the critical bits of knowledge and rules that have unfurled in our investigation, giving an exhaustive outline of the comprehensive mending scene inside the setting of multispeciality medical clinics.

1. All encompassing Mending as a Change in outlook:

    At its center, Comprehensive Mending addresses a takeoff from reductionist medical services models, stressing a sweeping way to deal with patient consideration. It implies a change in perspective from the separated treatment of side effects to a more significant comprehension of the interconnected idea of wellbeing. The all encompassing methodology perceives that ideal prosperity can't be accomplished by tending to one part of wellbeing in segregation yet requires a complete comprehension and coordination of physical, mental, profound, and otherworldly components.

2. Multispeciality Clinics as Centers of All encompassing Recuperating:

    Multispeciality emergency clinics act as the focal points where the all encompassing recuperating worldview flourishes and twists. These establishments typify the combination of different clinical strengths, cultivating cooperative and interdisciplinary ways to deal with patient consideration. The extensive idea of multispeciality clinics positions them as ideal settings for the combination of all encompassing standards, perceiving that the intricacies of wellbeing require an aggregate and facilitated exertion from different clinical disciplines.

3. Verifiable Viewpoints and Development:

Our investigation ventured through the Verifiable Viewpoints on Comprehensive Medication, uncovering the underlying foundations of all encompassing mending in antiquated customs that perceived the interconnectedness of brain, body, and soul. The Advancement of Multispeciality Emergency clinics further uncovered the movement from specific clinical practices to coordinated medical care models. This verifiable setting established the groundwork for the contemporary comprehension that all encompassing mending is definitely not an original idea yet a reintegration of old insight into present day clinical practices.

4. Incorporating Customary and Current Medication:

The Incorporation of Customary and Current Medication arose as a basic subject, underscoring that comprehensive mending doesn't nullify the worth of present day clinical intercessions yet looks to coordinate them flawlessly with conventional and integral methodologies. The concurrence of proof based medication and elective treatments inside multispeciality emergency clinics exhibits a guarantee to giving patients a range of care choices that line up with their inclinations and comprehensive prosperity.

5. Groundworks of All encompassing Recuperating:

The Groundworks of All encompassing Recuperating lie in a profound comprehension of the interconnectedness of psyche, body, and soul. This central rule guides experts in fitting mediations that go past side effect the board, tending to the underlying drivers of wellbeing challenges. The comprehensive methodology recognizes the impact of way of life, climate, and individual convictions on wellbeing results, encouraging a patient-focused model that thinks about the whole of a singular's prosperity.

6. Meaning of Multispeciality Medical clinics:

The Meaning of Multispeciality Medical clinics in All encompassing Recuperating reaches out past their job as therapy focuses. These organizations are impetuses for cooperative exploration, interdisciplinary joint effort, and the reconciliation of creative innovations. The all encompassing worldview flourishes in the dynamic and various climate of multispeciality medical clinics, where specific skill merges to give a comprehensive, patient-driven way to deal with medical care.

7. Exhaustive Patient Consideration:

Far reaching Patient Consideration arose as a focal principle, stressing that comprehensive mending stretches out past clinical medicines to include the general prosperity of patients. Cooperation Among Claims to fame guarantees that patients get incorporated and composed care, perceiving that tending to the different necessities of people requires a synergistic exertion from experts across different disciplines.

8. Comprehensive Way to deal with Finding and Treatment:
The Comprehensive Way to deal with Finding and Therapy highlights the significance of thinking about the entire individual in clinical evaluations and mediations. By perceiving the interconnected idea of physical and psychological well-being, professionals can tailor demonstrative and treatment designs that line up with the comprehensive recuperating worldview. This approach adds to a more significant comprehension of wellbeing difficulties and cultivates customized mediations that address the remarkable necessities of every person.

9. Establishing a Mending Climate:
Establishing a Mending Climate and Planning Patient-Accommodating Spaces recognizes the effect of the actual climate on profound prosperity. The plan and climate inside multispeciality medical clinics assume a vital part in cultivating a feeling of solace, serenity, and recuperating. These drives add to a comprehensive patient encounter that goes past clinical medicines to include the general recuperating venture.

10. Incorporating Elective Treatments:

Coordinating Elective Treatments perceives the worth of correlative modalities in improving all encompassing mending. From care rehearses and expressive expressions treatments to energy medication and integrative sustenance, these treatments add to a more extensive and patient-focused approach. Multispeciality medical clinics effectively embrace these other options, offering patients a range of decisions that line up with their all encompassing prosperity.

9.2 Call to Action for Healthcare Institutions

Source of inspiration for Medical services Establishments: Embracing Comprehensive Recuperating for an Extraordinary Future

Following our broad investigation into the domains of Comprehensive Recuperating in Multispeciality Emergency clinics, a resonating source of inspiration arises — a call that moves medical services foundations to rise above traditional limits and embrace an all encompassing worldview that tends to the sum of human prosperity. As we stand at the junction of conventional clinical practices and the groundbreaking capability of comprehensive recuperating, a convincing basic emerges for medical care organizations to support this change in outlook. This source of inspiration is a clarion require a significant change in the manner medical care is conceptualized, conveyed, and experienced.

1. Coordination of Comprehensive Standards into Center Medical care Models:
The most vital phase in noting this source of inspiration is the joining of all encompassing standards into the center models of medical care establishments.

This requires a change in outlook — from review wellbeing as an assortment of segregated side effects to perceiving the interconnected idea of physical, mental, close to home, and otherworldly prosperity. Medical care organizations should effectively integrate comprehensive methods of reasoning into their statements of purpose, smart courses of action, and functional systems. The reconciliation of comprehensive recuperating ought to be woven into the texture of hierarchical culture, directing dynamic cycles at each level.

2. Foundation of Comprehensive Recuperating Focuses inside Establishments:
   To really support comprehensive recuperating, medical services organizations ought to think about the foundation of devoted All encompassing Mending Places inside their premises. These focuses would act as centers for the joining of conventional and corresponding treatments, care practices, and patient training programs. By assigning explicit spaces for all encompassing recuperating, organizations signal a promise to furnishing patients with a far reaching range of care choices that stretch out past customary clinical intercessions. These focuses become central focuses for cooperative examination, interdisciplinary coordinated effort, and the development of a recuperating climate.

3. Persistent Schooling and Preparing for Medical care Experts:
   The fruitful execution of comprehensive mending requires a labor force that is knowledgeable in its standards and practices. Medical services foundations ought to put resources into persistent schooling and preparing programs for their experts, guaranteeing that professionals across different claims to fame are prepared to embrace and coordinate all encompassing methodologies into their consideration conveyance. This instructive drive ought to incorporate clinical perspectives as well as the way of thinking and ethos of all encompassing mending, cultivating a social shift toward a patient-focused and complete medical care model.

4. Research Drives to Approve and Progress All encompassing Methodologies:
   The source of inspiration reaches out to the domain of exploration, encouraging medical services organizations to effectively participate in drives that approve and progress comprehensive methodologies. This includes supporting exploration projects that investigate the viability of comprehensive mediations, the effect of way of life and natural variables on wellbeing, and the combination of conventional and current recuperating modalities. By adding to the collection of proof supporting all encompassing recuperating, foundations assume a significant part in molding the future direction of medical care and laying out comprehensive practices as vital parts of standard medication.

5. Joint effort Among Strengths and Disciplines:
   Joint effort Among Strengths isn't simply an idea; a source of inspiration orders separating storehouses and cultivating interdisciplinary cooperation inside medical care establishments. This cooperation reaches out past customary clinical disciplines to incorporate specialists of elective treatments, nutritionists,

psychological well-being experts, and comprehensive mending specialists. The collaboration among different fortes makes an all encompassing environment where the aggregate skill of different disciplines unites to give far reaching and patient-focused care.

6. Interest in Creative Advancements for All encompassing Medical services:
Medical care establishments are asked to put resources into inventive innovations that upgrade the conveyance of all encompassing medical services. This includes the combination of man-made reasoning for customized medication, high level imaging advancements for precise diagnostics, and telemedicine stages for distant patient commitment. By utilizing state of the art innovations, organizations work on the effectiveness of medical care conveyance as well as improve the openness of comprehensive administrations to a more extensive populace.

7. Promotion for Strategy Changes and Repayment Designs:
The source of inspiration reaches out past institutional limits to advocate for strategy changes and repayment structures that perceive and uphold all encompassing mending. Medical services foundations ought to effectively take part in backing endeavors to impact medical care arrangements, empowering the consideration of all encompassing methodologies in standard consideration conventions. Moreover, upholding for changes in repayment structures guarantees that all encompassing mediations are monetarily reasonable, cultivating a feasible model for organizations to integrate these practices into their standard contributions.

8. Development of Patient-Driven and Enabling Practices:
At the core of comprehensive recuperating is the strengthening of patients to effectively partake in their prosperity. Medical services establishments ought to develop patient-driven rehearses that focus on shared independent direction, individualized care plans, and patient training. This includes making stages for open correspondence, furnishing patients with devices for self-administration, and cultivating a medical care climate where people feel appreciated, regarded, and effectively engaged with their mending process.

9. Center around Preventive Medical services and Local area Wellbeing:
The source of inspiration stretches out past the limits of clinic walls to underscore a proactive spotlight on preventive medical care and local area wellbeing. Medical services organizations ought to put resources into local area outreach programs, wellbeing instruction drives, and preventive consideration systems that address the underlying drivers of wellbeing challenges. By embracing a populace wellbeing the executives approach, establishments become heroes of local area prosperity, adding to the production of better social orders.

10. Obligation to Moral and Comprehensive Practices:

A vital part of the source of inspiration is a pledge to moral and comprehensive practices. Medical care organizations are encouraged to maintain the standards of honesty, straightforwardness, and inclusivity in their all encompassing recuperating tries. This includes guaranteeing that comprehensive methodologies are grounded in proof based works on, advancing social ability, and recognizing the different necessities and inclinations of patients. Moral contemplations ought to direct every part of the comprehensive recuperating venture, from research drives to patient consideration conveyance.

9.3 The Future Landscape of Holistic Healthcare

The Future Scene of Comprehensive Medical services: Exploring a Change in perspective in Wellbeing

As we peer into the future, the scene of medical services is going through an extraordinary development, impelled by the combination of comprehensive standards and the acknowledgment of the interconnected idea of human prosperity. The excursion toward an all encompassing medical care worldview isn't simply a hypothetical idea however a substantial shift that is reshaping the manner in which people see and experience health. This investigation dives into the expected eventual fate of all encompassing medical services, imagining a scene that focuses on complete, patient-focused, and interconnected ways to deal with prosperity.

1. Customized and Accuracy All encompassing Medication:
   One of the signs representing things to come scene of all encompassing medical services is the union of customized and accuracy medication inside a comprehensive structure. As headways in genomics, proteomics, and other sub-atomic sciences keep on unfurling, medical care experts will have phenomenal admittance to individualized information. This abundance of data will take into consideration the fitting of comprehensive mediations in view of an individual's extraordinary hereditary cosmetics, way of life factors, and natural impacts. Accuracy all encompassing medication will arise as a foundation, enhancing remedial procedures to completely address the particular requirements of every person.

2. Mechanical Headways in All encompassing Medical services:
   The future scene of comprehensive medical services is complicatedly interwoven with innovative headways that improve availability, productivity, and the general patient experience. Telemedicine, augmented reality, and man-made consciousness will assume significant parts in expanding comprehensive consideration past customary medical care settings. Patients will approach virtual wellbeing stages, customized wellbeing applications, and ongoing teleconsultations, encouraging consistent commitment to their all encompassing prosperity. Wearable innovations will develop to screen actual wellbeing boundaries as well as variables connected with mental and close to home wellbeing, giving a more all encompassing and continuous comprehension of a singular's wellbeing.

3. Preventive Medical services and All encompassing Health Projects:
    A critical shift toward preventive medical care and comprehensive wellbeing
    projects will portray the future scene. Medical care establishments will progres-
    sively underscore proactive procedures that address the main drivers of well-
    being challenges, zeroing in on way of life alterations, sustenance, and mental
    prosperity. All encompassing wellbeing projects will stretch out past receptive
    intercessions to engage people with the information and devices for keeping up
    with ideal wellbeing. These projects will be custom-made to assorted populaces,
    advancing inclusivity and tending to wellbeing abberations.

4. Interdisciplinary Cooperation and All encompassing Reconciliation:
    The fate of all encompassing medical services will observer a reinforcing of inter-
    disciplinary coordinated effort, separating storehouses between clinical claims
    to fame and encouraging comprehensive joining. Medical services organizations
    will lay out cooperative consideration groups containing experts from assorted
    disciplines, including doctors, attendants, emotional wellness professionals, nu-
    tritionists, and elective treatment specialists. This cooperative methodology will
    guarantee that patients get extensive consideration that addresses the physical,
    mental, close to home, and profound components of their prosperity.

5. Comprehensive Recuperating Focuses and Integrative Medication Divisions:
    The foundation of devoted All encompassing Recuperating Focuses and In-
    tegrative Medication Divisions inside medical services establishments will turn
    out to be more common later on scene. These specific habitats will act as central
    focuses for the reconciliation of conventional and corresponding treatments,
    care rehearses, and comprehensive schooling. Patients will have the choice to get
    care that consistently consolidates customary clinical mediations with elective
    modalities, making a cooperative energy that tends to the diverse idea of well-
    being challenges.

6. Mind-Body-Soul Association in Medical services:
    The acknowledgment of the psyche body-soul association will be a core value
    later on scene of comprehensive medical services. Medical care professionals will
    progressively recognize the effect of mental and profound prosperity on actual
    wellbeing, prompting a more coordinated approach in finding and therapy. Care
    practices, contemplation, and other comprehensive mediations that encourage
    profound prosperity will be incorporated into care plans, perceiving that genu-
    ine health envelops amicability across all elements of human experience.

7. Comprehensive Restoration and Psychological wellness Backing:
    Comprehensive ways to deal with restoration and emotional well-being backing
    will become norm in store for medical care. Restoration projects will go past
    non-intrusive treatments to incorporate mental and profound prosperity drives,
    perceiving the interconnectedness of recuperation. Emotional well-being back-
    ing will be consistently coordinated into essential consideration, and elective

treatments like workmanship treatment, music treatment, and care based mediations will assume necessary parts in advancing mental health.

8. Comprehensive Nursing Practices:
The job of nursing later on scene of comprehensive medical services will be raised, with an emphasis on All encompassing Nursing Practices. Attendants will be prepared to incorporate all encompassing standards into their consideration conveyance, tending to the actual parts of wellbeing as well as the close to home and profound necessities of patients. Patient schooling, guiding, and the advancement of taking care of oneself practices will be fundamental parts of comprehensive nursing, cultivating a cooperative and enabling medical services climate.

9. Worldwide Wellbeing Joint effort and All encompassing Points of view:
The fate of all encompassing medical care will observer expanded worldwide wellbeing coordinated effort, with medical care foundations embracing comprehensive viewpoints from assorted social and customary practices. Incorporating conventional recuperating techniques from different societies into standard medical services will turn into a foundation of comprehensive and patient-focused care. This worldwide trade of all encompassing information will improve medical services works on, giving a more far reaching comprehension of wellbeing that rises above geological limits.

10. Patient Strengthening and Dynamic Support:

A central part representing things to come scene of comprehensive medical care is the strengthening of patients to effectively take part in their prosperity. Patients will be urged to be accomplices in their consideration, effectively captivating in dynamic cycles and taking on proactive way of life decisions. All encompassing medical care suppliers will stress patient training, advancing a more profound comprehension of the interconnected idea of wellbeing and the job of people in their own comprehensive prosperity.

www.ingramcontent.com/pod-product-compliance
Lightning Source LLC
LaVergne TN
LVHW050642200726
843506LV00010B/1331